In 2000, over 68% of American women were breastfeeding newborns. But only 31.4% were still nursing by their babies' sixth month, and only 17.6% by their first birthday.

Based on the latest research and the American Academy of Pediatrics' Policy on Breastfeeding, this essential handbook answers new mothers' most common questions about breast-feeding, including:

- How will I know if my baby is getting enough milk?
- What kind of diet is best while breastfeeding?
- Is my baby latched-on properly?
- Will I be able to breastfeed once I return to work?
- How can I keep my partner involved while I breastfeed?
- How can I get friends and family to support this important decision?
- How do I breastfeed a teething toddler?
- At what age do I wean my child—and how?
- Can I still breastfeed after breast surgery?
- Will taking aspirin or other medications adversely affect my breastfeeding baby?

. . . and much more, to help you and your baby get the health-iest possible start. The benefits will last a lifetime.

Child Care Books from
the American Academy of Pediatrics

Caring for Your Baby and Young Child:
Birth to Age 5

Caring for Your School-Age Child:
Ages 5 to 12

Caring for Your Teenager:
Ages 12 to 21

Guide to Your Child's Nutrition

Guide to Your Child's Allergies and Asthma

Guide to Your Child's Sleep

Guide to Your Child's Symptoms

Your Baby's First Year

American Academy of Pediatrics

New Mother's Guide to Breastfeeding

Joan Younger Meek, M.D.,
M.S., R.D., FAAP, IBCLC,
Editor-in-Chief
with Sherill Tippins

BANTAM BOOKS

AMERICAN ACADEMY OF PEDIATRICS NEW MOTHER'S GUIDE TO BREASTFEEDING

A Bantam Book published by arrangement with the
American Academy of Pediatrics / August 2002

Book design by Lynn Newmark

Library of Congress Cataloging-in-Publication Data

American Academy of Pediatrics new mother's guide to breastfeeding /
Joan Younger Meek, editor-in-chief, with Sherill Tippins.
p.   cm.
Includes bibliographical references and index.
ISBN 0-553-38107-5
1. Breast feeding. 1. Title: New mother's guide to breastfeeding.
II. Meek, Joan Younger. III. Tippins, Sherill. IV. American Academy of
Pediatrics.
RJ216.A477 2002
649'.33—dc21   2002023885

Published simultaneously in the United States and Canada

PRINTED IN THE UNITED STATES OF AMERICA

RRH 10   9   8   7   6   5   4   3   2   1

REVIEWERS/CONTRIBUTORS

Editor-in-Chief
Joan Younger Meek, M.D., M.S., R.D., FAAP, IBCLC

AAP Board of Directors Reviewer
Kathryn Piziali Nichol, M.D., M.S., FAAP

American Academy of Pediatrics

Executive Director
Joe M. Sanders, Jr., M.D., FAAP

Associate Executive Director
Roger F. Suchyta, M.D., FAAP

Director, Department of Education
Robert Perelman, M.D., FAAP

Director, Division of Public Education
Lisa R. Miller

Manager, Consumer Publishing
Division of Public Education
Brent L. Heathcott, CAE

Coordinator, Consumer Publishing
Division of Public Education
Veronica Laude Noland

Director, Department of Community Pediatrics
Thomas F. Tonniges, M.D.

Director, Division of Community Health Services
Laura D. Aird, M.S.

DEDICATION

This book is dedicated to all the people who recognize that children are our greatest inspiration in the present and our greatest hope for the future.

The American Academy of Pediatrics recognizes that breastfeeding is important for the optimal health and development of infants and children. This publication was developed in gratitude to those mothers and professionals who have preserved breastfeeding in our culture and in the hope that increasing numbers of women in present and future generations will experience this unique opportunity to both nourish and nurture their children. It is our desire that women who read this book will find encouragement to make the decision to breastfeed, help for the early breastfeeding days, practical solutions for breastfeeding challenges, resources to help meet their personal goals for breastfeeding, and support to continue breastfeeding for as long as they choose.

From Joan Younger Meek, editor-in-chief:
With personal thanks to Sandy T., for her mother-to-mother support in encouraging me to breastfeed; to Katie, Rachel, and Joseph, for teaching me how to be a breastfeeding mother; to Joshua, for teaching me how to solve breastfeeding challenges; to Dr. Deborah Squire, for showing me how to be a breastfeeding-supportive pediatrician; and to the many babies and families who have taught me the joys of breastfeeding.

TABLE OF CONTENTS

Foreword

The American Academy of Pediatrics (AAP) welcomes you to the *New Mother's Guide to Breastfeeding,* the latest in its series of parenting books.

Deciding to breastfeed is one of the most important decisions a mother-to-be can make to give her newborn the best possible start in life. Even so, many women have questions and concerns about breastfeeding and want to know why breastfeeding is so beneficial. This book will help mothers and fathers understand the neurological, psychological, and immunological benefits of human milk; prepare for breastfeeding before a baby is born; plan for the first feeding and bringing the baby home; understand the father's role in breastfeeding; continue breastfeeding if the mother returns to work; and so much more.

What separates this book from other reference books on breastfeeding is that pediatricians who specialize in this area have reviewed it extensively. Under the direction of our editor-in-chief, the material in this book was developed with the assistance of numerous reviewers and contributors from the American Academy of Pediatrics. Because medical information is constantly changing, every effort has been made to ensure that this book contains the most up-to-date findings. Readers may want to visit the AAP Website at www.aap.org to keep current on this and other subjects. Parents can also access consumer health information from the AAP at www.medem.com, an e-health network created by the AAP and other leading medical societies.

It is our hope that this book will become an invaluable resource and reference guide for parents. We are confident that parents and caregivers will find the book extremely helpful. We encourage its use in concert with the advice and counsel of our readers' pediatricians, who will provide individual guidance and assistance related to the health of children.

The AAP is an organization of fifty-five thousand primary-care pediatricians, pediatric medical subspecialists, and pediatric surgical specialists dedicated to the health, safety, and well-being of infants, children, adolescents, and young adults. The *New Mother's Guide to Breastfeeding* is part of the Academy's ongoing educational efforts to provide parents and caregivers with high-quality information on a broad spectrum of children's health issues.

Joe M. Sanders, Jr., M.D., FAAP
Executive Director

CHAPTER 1

Choosing to Breastfeed

"Nursing my daughter was a decision I made even before she was conceived. I was not breastfed as a child but had seen with other parents the bond that breastfeeding brings to the mother–child relationship. I also understood the nutritional and immunologic benefits that mother's milk provides the infant and wanted the very best for my child."

—Stacy, 31, mother of Adam

With three weeks remaining until her baby's due date, Vicki could hardly wait for the day to arrive. She and her husband had completed their natural-childbirth course and toured the hospital where their baby would be born. They had baby clothes ready and had even bought their first supply of diapers. Yet as Vicki focused on tying up loose ends at work prior to her maternity leave, she couldn't help feeling nervous about some aspects of new motherhood. *Will I be able to breastfeed?* she wondered. *My cousin tried, but she quit after a week. And what about when I start working again?* she asked herself as she packed a box of papers to take home. *The baby will have to use a bottle then. Should I start him on formula so he doesn't have to switch later on?*

Suddenly weary, Vicki sat down and rested a hand on her stomach. Feeling a slow, rolling movement beneath her hand, she looked down with a wan smile. "I want the best for you," she said to her baby. "I just wish I had someone to teach me about this. What's really important for your health, and how can I make sure you get it?"

DOES BREASTFEEDING MAKE SENSE FOR ME?

If you, too, are about to give birth, you may share Vicki's concerns or have other urgent questions about how, when, and even whether you should breastfeed your child. The act of nursing—one of nature's most rewarding and beneficial processes—can sometimes seem intimidating when you face a host of other commitments and hear a great deal of conflicting advice. In the following chapters, you will find clear answers to many of these questions, solutions to your problems, and information about the array of breastfeeding support services—hospital nurses, pediatricians, obstetricians, family physicians, lactation specialists, and breastfeeding support groups—that are in place to help mothers breastfeed their children successfully.

Such efforts have been made because an enormous amount of research demonstrates how beneficial breastfeeding is for babies. We now know that nursing your child not only strengthens the quality of your relationship with her but improves her health, enhances her brain development, and provides her with precisely the type of nourishment she needs at each critical stage of her development. The benefits of human breastmilk so greatly exceed that of any alternative method of infant feeding, in fact, that health organizations around the globe have united to promote this natural source of

Breastfeeding ensures the healthiest start to an infant's life and provides important benefits for both mother and baby.

nutritional and emotional sustenance for babies. The World Health Organization (WHO), for example, encourages women to breastfeed exclusively for six months and to continue to breastfeed for at least two years to take advantage of human milk's ability to provide the best nutrition and protect against infection. The American Academy of Pediatrics (AAP) recommends exclusive breastfeeding (no water, formula, other liquids, or solids) for about the first six months of life, followed by breastfeeding with the introduction of solid foods for the next six months, and continued breastfeeding thereafter as long as mutually desired by mother and baby.

Where We Stand

As the United States' foremost association of board-certified pediatricians, the American Academy of Pediatrics is committed to improving the health of all children. We recognize breastfeeding's role in creating the best possible health, developmental, and psychosocial outcomes for the infant. Therefore, we recommend breastfeeding as the sole source of nutrition for infants for about the first six months; breastfeeding in combination with solid foods through at least twelve months; and continued breastfeeding thereafter for as long as mutually desired by mother and baby. While the ultimate decision to breastfeed is yours, it is our responsibility to provide you with complete, up-to-date information on the benefits and methods of breastfeeding to ensure that your feeding decision is a fully informed one. (For more information about the AAP's breastfeeding recommendations and policies, please log on to the AAP Website at www.aap.org.)

As you prepare for motherhood, you will want answers to *all* of your questions about breastfeeding. You will want to consider how it is possible to combine breastfeeding with work outside the home, how you can fully involve your partner* in parenting a breastfed infant, and how to adjust if breastfeeding doesn't begin smoothly. You will need to understand how breastfeeding works so you can feel assured that certain behaviors are normal or recognize any difficulties. Finally, you will want to find knowledgeable breastfeeding support services in your area.

As pediatricians, we want to share all we know to help you. With this guide, we will provide information, encouragement, and support as you learn this vital new skill. We will show you how many millions of women—working outside the home or not, married or not, first-time or experienced mothers—have provided the best for their babies through breastfeeding, and how you can too.

DID MY MOTHER BREASTFEED?

When you were an infant you may not have been breastfed, though your mother may have been and your grandmother was even more likely to have been breastfed. Breastfeeding, like many other techniques for nurturing children, has passed in and out of fashion according to parenting trends, society's needs, and the accumulation of reliable research.

Of course, few alternatives were available to mothers a century ago. In the early 1900s, the majority of American women breastfed their infants, and over half of the babies were still being breastfed beyond the first year of life. Mothers who could not or chose not to breastfeed used a wet nurse, fed animal milk to their babies, or made do with crude mixtures of flour, rice, and water called "pap." The newborns' chances of survival decreased significantly as a result. During the decades that followed, however,

* Please note that we use *partner* and *your baby's father* interchangeably to respect the relationship you are in.

glass bottles and rubber nipples became more widely available and pasteurization and vitamin supplementation more common-place. As a result, alternatives to breastfeeding became more practical and prevalent, though almost nothing was known about how these artificial infant feedings affected children's long-term health and development. During World War II, as more women worked outside the home, formula feeding increased even more and continued to increase through the 1950s and 1960s. By 1966, only eighteen percent of babies were being breastfed at the time they *left the hospital*, and this percentage dropped sharply soon after the babies arrived home. In the early 1970s in the United States, breastfeeding rates hit a record low.

At about this time, however, medical research began to reveal new truths about the advantages of mother's milk for infant health and development. Scientists noted that babies who breast-fed were more resistant to diseases in the environment. They caught fewer colds, suffered from fewer ear infections, and expe-rienced fewer allergies. Even their mothers appeared to recover from childbirth more quickly and easily. Such findings, along with the mid-seventies movement toward a more natural child-birth and parenting experience, caused breastfeeding rates to begin climbing again. In 1982, nearly sixty-two percent of new-borns were nourished by their mother's milk after birth. By 2000, this number had increased to more than sixty-eight percent. Un-fortunately, work conflicts and lack of support caused many mothers to give up nursing quite early, and this continues to be the case. Of the American newborns breastfed in 2000, only about thirty-one percent were still nursing by their sixth month, and less than eighteen percent by their first birthday. Yet studies keep revealing the fascinating ways in which the content of breastmilk changes to suit the baby at every stage of develop-ment, continuing to provide precisely the developmental, psy-chological, and health benefits a baby needs through the first year and beyond.

Today, mothers are not forced to choose between only two al-ternatives—breastfeeding their babies or giving them formula.

They may opt to breastfeed their babies directly; provide them with bottles of breastmilk that they have expressed and stored for later use; obtain donated, processed breastmilk from a milk bank when their own milk production is insufficient or their milk cannot be used; or use commercially produced formula available in supermarkets and pharmacies as either a supplement to their own breastmilk or a replacement for breastfeeding. Which option you choose at any particular time will depend on your circumstances and you and your baby's needs. However, before you make your decision, you owe it to your baby to learn how breastfeeding benefits you both. Consider the support services (lactation specialists, breastfeeding support groups, and on-line information), efficient aids to breastfeeding (breast pumps, breastmilk-storage containers), and increased social acceptance (more breastfeeding in public, maternity leave, private rooms provided at work for nursing mothers) now available to help you succeed. It is our hope that as you read about breastfeeding's benefits for your baby and consider how nursing can be a part of your life, you will decide to give breastfeeding a try. After all, babies are not babies for very long. They deserve the healthiest start they can get.

WHY IS BREASTFEEDING SO GOOD FOR MY BABY?

Formula for babies has become such a pervasive part of our culture that many people assume it must be as good for babies as human milk. After all, formula is designed to contain many of the nutrients provided in breastmilk—and babies who are fed formula clearly grow and develop adequately. Yet the fact remains that human milk and infant formula differ in a number of fundamental ways. Breastmilk is such a rich, nourishing mixture that scientists have yet to identify all of its elements; no formula manufacturer has managed or will ever be able to fully replicate it.

◆ IMMUNOLOGIC BENEFITS

Human milk provides virtually all the protein, sugar, and fat your baby needs to be healthy, and it also contains many substances that benefit your baby's immune system, including antibodies, immune factors, enzymes, and white blood cells. These substances protect your baby against a wide variety of diseases and infections not only while he is breastfeeding but in some cases long after he has weaned. Formula cannot offer this protection.

If you develop a cold while breastfeeding, for example, you are likely to pass the cold germs on to your baby—but the antibodies your body produces to fight that cold will also be passed on, through your breastmilk. These antibodies will help your infant conquer the cold germs quickly and effectively and possibly avoid developing the cold altogether. This defense against illnesses significantly decreases the chances that your breastfeeding baby will suffer from ear infections, vomiting, diarrhea, pneumonia, urinary-tract infections, or certain types of spinal meningitis. Even infants in group child-care programs, who tend to catch more germs due to their close proximity, are less likely to become ill if they are breastfed or fed bottled breastmilk that their mothers have expressed.

Allergists recommend breastfeeding as a way to decrease the risk of developing food allergies and eczema in families prone to these conditions. Human breastmilk contains human milk proteins, not the proteins of cow's milk or soy milk, which are "foreign" to the baby's immune system and may stimulate an allergic response. Transfer of the mother's antibodies and other immunologic substances may also explain why children who breastfeed for more than six months are less likely to contract childhood acute leukemia than those who receive formula. Studies have demonstrated a reduced risk of Sudden Infant Death Syndrome (SIDS) among babies who breastfeed, though the reasons for this are not fully understood. Recent research even indicates that breastfed infants are less likely to be obese in later life and that breastfed daughters are at reduced risk of developing breast cancer as adults.

HEALTH RISKS FOR FORMULA-FED VS. BREASTFED BABIES

A formula-fed baby has _____ the chance of contracting
_____ as a breastfed baby during the breastfeeding
period:

2 to 7 times	allergies, eczema
3 times	ear infections
3 times	gastroenteritis
3.8 times	meningitis
2.6 to 5.5 times	urinary-tract infections
2.4 times	diabetes, type 1
2 times	Sudden Infant Death Syndrome (SIDS)
1.7 to 5 times	pneumonia/lower-respiratory-tract infection
1.5 to 1.9 times	inflammatory bowel disease
1 to 6.7 times	Hodgkin's lymphoma

Adapted from: *American Family Physician,* April 1, 2000, Vol. 61, No. 7.

◆ BREASTMILK AND INFANT DEVELOPMENT

In addition to changing to defend against threats in the environment, the composition of human milk also adjusts over time to meet your child's needs at each stage of development—with the greatest changes occurring in the critical first few weeks after your infant is born. The first milk your body produces, called colostrum, is low in volume but high in protein and easy for a newborn to digest. (If you deliver prematurely, your colostrum will contain even more protein and different types of fats that are important for premature babies.) After birth, colostrum gradually gives way to more mature milk, which is much greater in volume, lower in protein, and higher in lactose and fat, in accordance with your infant's evolving needs. The fat content of human milk changes during the course of a single feeding—

starting out low in fat and increasing until the end of the feeding. The composition of mother's milk even changes over the course of the day.

The fatty acids found in breastmilk are, in part, responsible for its ability to facilitate optimal brain development. An increasing number of studies show that scores on IQ and other cognitive-ability tests of children who were breastfed as infants are higher than those of children who were fed formula, independent of socioeconomic factors or the mother's intelligence score. This increase is particularly striking among low-birthweight infants. Of course, breastfeeding alone does not guarantee that your baby will be a child prodigy. But the evidence shows that in many aspects of infant development a mother's milk does offer the child an *early advantage* that formula doesn't. Because a baby's brain develops at its most rapid rate during infancy and early childhood, the specific types of fat in breastmilk are important for developing the connections that enable brain cells to communicate with one another.

◆ PSYCHOLOGICAL BENEFITS

Your newborn also benefits from the physical closeness of nursing. Thrust from the close, dark womb into an overwhelming experience of bright lights, loud noises, and new smells, your baby needs the reassurance of your continued physical presence. By holding him safe in your arms and giving nourishment from your body, you offer him a sense of continuity from pre- to post-birth life. Gazing into your eyes, your baby comes to understand that he is loved and protected and that you are there to provide for his needs as he adjusts to this new world. This emotional bond is as vital as the nutritional benefit he receives from you. Scientists now tell us that infants learn best in a context of emotional closeness with an adult. Breastfeeding promotes a growing attachment between the two of you that will continue to play an important role in your baby's development for years to come.

IS BREASTFEEDING GOOD FOR ME TOO?

Breastfeeding is a wonderful gift for both you and your baby. Many mothers feel fulfillment and joy from the physical and emotional communion they experience with their child while nursing. These feelings are augmented by the release of the hormones prolactin, which produces a peaceful, nurturing sensation that allows you to relax and focus on your child, and oxytocin, which promotes a strong sense of love and attachment between the two of you. These pleasant feelings may be one of the reasons so many women who have breastfed their first child choose to breastfeed the children who follow.

Breastfeeding provides health benefits for mothers in addition to emotional satisfaction. Overall, women who breastfeed tend to lose pregnancy weight more quickly—usually at a rate of about one or two pounds per month. The hormone oxytocin acts to return the uterus to its regular size more quickly and can reduce postpartum bleeding. Studies show that women who have breastfed experience reduced rates of ovarian cancer and breast cancer later in life. Some studies suggest that breastfeeding may lead to an increase in bone mineral density after weaning that can protect you against osteoporosis and bone fractures in older age, although this has not been proven conclusively. Finally, exclusive breastfeeding delays the return of the mother's menstrual period, which can help extend the time between pregnancies. (Exclusive breastfeeding can provide a natural form of contraception if the mother's menses have not returned, the baby is breastfeeding day and night, and the baby is less than six months old. See Chapter 6 for more information about breastfeeding and birth control.)

There are quite a few practical advantages to breastfeeding as well—bonuses the entire family can appreciate. For example, human milk is much less expensive than formula. During nursing you will need, at most, an extra three hundred to five hundred calories daily to produce sufficient breastmilk for your baby, while formula costs three or more dollars per day. At night, putting a baby to your breast is much simpler and faster than getting up to prepare or warm a bottle of formula. (Your partner can make night feedings even easier by changing the baby and bringing her to you for nursing.) It's wonderful, too, to be able to pick up the baby and go out—whether around town or on longer trips—without having to carry a bag full of feeding equipment. Breastfeeding is also good for the environment, since there are no bottles to wash or formula cans to throw away.

As welcome as all of these benefits are, though, most mothers put the feeling of maternal fulfillment at the top of their list of reasons for breastfeeding. Breastfeeding provides a unique emotional experience for the nursing mother and the baby. Your partner, the baby's siblings, and other relatives can all appreciate the new member of the family being welcomed in such a loving way.

IS FORMULA AN OPTION?

As scientists learn more about the composition of human breastmilk, makers of formula continue to refine their product in an attempt to simulate its attributes as closely as possible. It is impossible to perfectly mimic a substance as complex as human breastmilk, but formula does provide an alternative in cases where it's not possible to breastfeed exclusively or to provide expressed or donated breastmilk in a bottle.

A small percentage of new mothers are affected by physical conditions that interfere with breastmilk production, such as insufficient development of the glands that produce milk (see Chapter 2) or the effects of breast-reduction surgery. In the U.S., women with HIV are advised not to breastfeed, since the virus may be passed to their infant in the milk. Mothers newly diagnosed with infectious tuberculosis should not breastfeed unless they are on medication. Breastfeeding is not advised while taking certain medications, and any medication you take while nursing should be approved by your doctor. If the medication is not recommended while breastfeeding, your doctor may be able to offer you a safer alternative. (See Chapter 5 for more information on medical conditions that may affect breastfeeding.)

The infant's medical condition, as well, may preclude breast-feeding. Some babies are unable to metabolize the sugar in human milk or cow's-milk-based formula due to a rare genetic disorder called galactosemia. (Most states test for this condition as part of the newborn-infant screen several days after birth.) Infants with the classic form of galactosemia must be fed a formula that does not contain lactose or milk sugar. Extremely premature infants may be unable to breastfeed initially and, in some instances, may require supplements along with breastmilk that their mothers have expressed.

While few clear medical issues prohibit breastfeeding, you may experience physical or psychological resistance to the process. Nursing your baby shouldn't hurt if your baby is attached (latched on) to the breast correctly, but incorrect attachment can cause nipple pain and even bleeding—particularly during the first few days of nursing. Some mothers feel discouraged by this negative early experience and are tempted to stop breastfeeding. However, in most cases, a hospital nurse, pediatrician, or lactation specialist can help you reposition your baby correctly at the breast and get nursing off to a much more comfortable start.

New mothers are also often strongly influenced by the advice and experiences of their female relatives and friends. If your mother or other women close to you did not breastfeed their children or do not understand its benefits, they may encourage you to forgo breastfeeding and feed your baby formula instead. Your baby's father may also advocate formula-feeding. In most cases these loved ones mean well but are not well-informed about the importance of breastfeeding. This book will provide you with answers to their questions or criticisms about breastfeeding and refer you to people in your community who will support whatever choice *you* make. If you find that you have become quite anxious about the breastfeeding experience—so much that your resistance may interfere with your relationship with your baby—

it may help to talk to experienced breastfeeding mothers to allay your fears.

Certainly, there is no reason to conclude that choosing any particular feeding plan makes you a good or a bad parent. Still, barring any definite medical or physical problems that would interfere with lactation, it is advantageous to breastfeed. If you and your baby stay focused on the process and you have a good support system in place, most breastfeeding problems can be resolved within the first few weeks so you can settle into a comfortable breastfeeding relationship.

While at least twelve months is ideal, any amount of breastfeeding provides important benefits for your baby. If you worry that you will not be able to breastfeed after you return to work, it's still quite worthwhile to breastfeed until then. As the time for returning to work or school approaches, you can experiment with using a breast pump, help your baby get used to taking expressed breastmilk from a bottle or alternative feeding method (see Chapter 9), and then reconsider whether it's really necessary to wean your child once you will be out of the house part of each day.

BREASTFEEDING: A NATURAL GIFT

Vicki's maternity leave finally began and she now eagerly counted down the days until her baby's birth. Only a week ago she sat in her office, worrying about whether or not she should breastfeed, but since then she had gathered a great deal of information on the topic to help her decide. Following the directions in a book about breastfeeding that she'd found at the library, she had checked with her doctor, contacted a local breastfeeding support group for advice, and talked with experienced friends about the logistics of nursing a baby while working. Her advisers encouraged her to talk to her boss about how she might find a private place for expressing breastmilk once she returned from maternity leave. To her surprise, her employer offered to make an

Q & A

How Will Breastfeeding Change My Life?

Q: *If I breastfeed, will I have to watch everything I eat, and do I have to drink milk all the time, as I did during pregnancy?*

A: In most cases you should maintain a healthy diet, as you would whether or not you were breastfeeding. (See Chapter 7 for more on nutrition.) One advantage of breastfeeding is that while you should eat an additional three hundred to five hundred calories per day, those calories add heft to your baby's thighs, not yours! You don't have to drink extra milk, since a breastfeeding mother's body efficiently absorbs calcium from other foods. In fact, you don't have to drink any cow's milk to make human milk. You do need a daily source of calcium in your diet, though, and will want to make sure your diet is adequate in vitamins and minerals. Consult your physician or your child's pediatrician if you're not sure that you are getting all the nutrients you need. A glass of wine or a cup of coffee is fine while nursing. In general, moderation is the key. In fact, a breastfeeding mother's diet is an excellent blueprint for a lifetime of healthy eating.

Q: *How can I manage to have free time to myself while breastfeeding on demand?*

A: During the first days after birth, all mothers, whether or not they breastfeed, must adjust to their babies' need for their almost constant presence. (This is usually not difficult, since you will want to get to know your baby and to rest and recuperate together.) Gradually, over the weeks that follow, you will find that you have an increasing amount of physical freedom. After the first few weeks, feedings will become more regular, giving you predictable times when you do not have to be present to breastfeed your child. With the proper preparation, your baby should be able to accept breastmilk that you've expressed ahead of time and left for him in a bottle, if you choose to do so. If you wait until breast-feeding is well established when your baby is at least three to four weeks old, this should not interfere with his ability to breastfeed. (See Chapter 9 for information on ways to prepare your baby to move from breast to bottle.) This is how many working mothers provide breastmilk for their babies, enjoying the closeness of breastfeeding when at home while still affording the health benefits of breastmilk when they're away. In short, breastfeeding promotes physical closeness with your baby but does not mean you are tied to him constantly.

Q: *How can my partner be an active, involved parent if I'm breastfeeding exclusively?*

A: Just as your partner has already played a vital co-parenting role by supporting you during pregnancy and will continue to do so during childbirth, his parenting role will remain crucial as your baby makes the *gradual* transition from attachment to your body toward interaction with others in his world. There are many ways to be a parent besides feeding the baby. Your partner can provide you with nutritious meals so you can better feed your infant, help with household chores so you can rest, play with the baby during awake time, and rock him to sleep by holding him against his chest and singing in a low, rumbling voice. If actually feeding the baby is important to your partner, he can offer your expressed breastmilk in a bottle after the baby is at least several weeks old and has fully adjusted to the breast. (In Chapter 9, this process will be presented in greater detail, and in Chapter 11 we offer suggestions on many more ways in which your partner can fully participate in the parenting experience.) The bottom line, though, is that each parent's gifts to his child are different, but all are equally valuable.

empty office available to her and even chatted for several minutes about how his wife had breastfed their baby and how beneficial he believed breastfeeding was. Vicki was relieved by his support.

Now that Vicki saw how it might be possible to nurse her baby for a longer period than she had thought, she was excited at the prospect of experiencing this special closeness with her baby. The decision to breastfeed had become a "no-brainer." She had talked to her obstetrician about her desire to breastfeed, had made an appointment with her child's pediatrician to discuss the practical aspects of breastfeeding, and had spoken with her husband about how he could help her adjust to nursing and share in parenting their baby. She had gone through her wardrobe, looking for shirts and blouses that could be easily pulled up or unbuttoned from the bottom up for breastfeeding. She had even taken a class on breastfeeding at her local hospital so she would know how to begin once her baby was born.

The following chapters are dedicated to helping you get ready for and experience your own breastfeeding journey, from preparing for those important early feedings to adjusting to home life, family life, and work life as a nursing mother and finally to moving with your child beyond breastfeeding. Hopefully, you will find that breastfeeding goes smoothly from the start. However, like anything new, it may take some time and practice to get the process going effectively. This is perfectly normal. In the meantime, stay positive and try not to get discouraged. Remember, your breastmilk will provide your baby with more than just food. Breastfeeding is a wonderful natural gift that only you can give your baby, and we hope you will discover it to be a rewarding experience for both of you.

CHAPTER 2

A Perfect Design:
How Breastfeeding Works

"It was so amazing, watching my body get ready to nourish this new baby. Everything she needed, my body was able to give. It made me think about what a powerful connection the mother–child bond really is, both before and after delivery."

—Tamara, 28, mother of Megan

Beatrice, thirty-seven, had long looked forward to having a child and, once she became pregnant, eagerly anticipated breastfeeding her baby daughter. Yet despite all her conversations about nursing with friends and relatives who were experienced mothers, several points about breastfeeding during the early months of breastfeeding came as a surprise. Beatrice wondered about the thick, yellow substance that her breasts produced for her baby during the first few days after childbirth, rather than the white milk she'd expected to see. "It's called colostrum," her friend told her. "It's this superconcentrated concoction that your body makes to feed your baby in the first few days."

After the colostrum had been replaced by more mature, bluish-white breastmilk, Beatrice was surprised to see the milk squirt out of a number of little holes in her nipples rather than in one steady stream. "You learn how it works pretty quickly," she commented months later. "Luckily, everything went smoothly for me and I managed to improvise even though I didn't understand much about how breastfeeding worked. If I had it to do again, though, I'd find out more about the process so I could tell the difference between what was normal and what wasn't. It sure would have put my mind more at ease."

PREPARING TO BREASTFEED

As you experience all of the physiological changes preceding the birth of your baby, which ones are preparing your body to breastfeed? And how does the process work? You probably noted early in your pregnancy—at around the fifth or sixth week—that your breasts had become fuller and your nipples were more tender than before. Your nipples and the darker-colored area around them, called the *areolae,* may have enlarged and darkened, and the small bumps on the areolae, called the *Montgomery's glands,* became

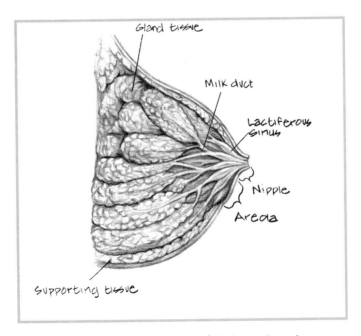

This schematic cross-section diagram of the breast shows that as your pregnancy progresses, the fatty and supportive tissues that normally make up most of the volume of the breast are replaced by glandular tissue necessary to produce milk.

more prominent. Starting about the third month of pregnancy, the complex interplay of a number of hormones—including prolactin, estrogen, progesterone, and human growth hormone— leads to the proliferation of milk ducts and gland-producing cells in your breasts as your body prepares for milk production.

As your pregnancy progresses, the glandular tissue necessary to produce milk replaces much of the fatty and supportive tissue that normally makes up most of the volume of your breast. This causes your breasts to become substantially larger during pregnancy and lactation. Such changes may worry you that breastfeeding will cause your breasts to sag or change shape after weaning, but there is no reason for concern. Once your baby is weaned from the breast (when you stop nursing and your milk glands are once again replaced by fatty and supportive tissue) and you return to your prepregnancy weight, your breasts will return to their approximate prepregnancy size and shape.

By the end of the second trimester, your body has become fully capable of producing breastmilk—which means that even if your child is born prematurely, you will be able to produce breastmilk. Colostrum, the first milk produced, is thick, somewhat sticky, and yellow or orange in color. (If you notice yellow or orange stains on the inside of your maternity bra, your breasts are making colostrum. However, some mothers do not notice any colostrum being secreted until after their babies are born.)

After your baby is born, the areolae of your breasts, and especially the nipples, will become exquisitely sensitive to touch. When your baby's mouth touches the nipple, nerve cells will send a signal to your brain, causing the release of the hormone oxytocin. Oxytocin causes tiny muscle cells within the breasts to contract, squeezing milk from the milk-producing cells down the milk ducts toward small sacs or sinuses near the nipples. As your baby suckles at the breast, drawing milk from the sinuses through the nipple and into her mouth, the production of oxytocin will increase, causing more milk to be moved through the ducts in a process called the *let-down* or *milk-ejection reflex*. This is a simplified description of the complex system by which your body ensures

A baby's mouth on its mother's nipple signals to the mother's brain
to release oxytocin, a hormone that causes the milk ducts to
contract and expel the milk, as well as causes the muscles of the
uterus to contract.

that whenever your infant is hungry, your body will provide her
with the nourishment she needs.

Many women who look forward to breastfeeding are concerned whether their breasts are large enough to provide milk for
their babies. While size may affect the volume of milk your
breasts can hold at any given time—so that you may need to
nurse more frequently if your breasts are smaller—breast size does
not determine how much milk you make overall. As long as your
baby is latched on and suckling correctly (see Chapter 4), the
amount of milk you produce is determined by how much your
baby nurses. The more milk she drinks, the more milk your body
will produce. The less she breastfeeds, the less milk produced.

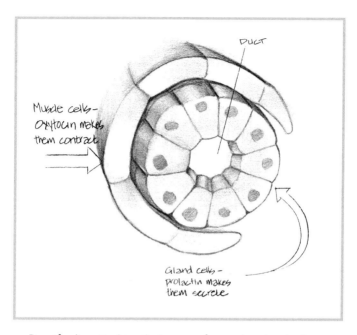

Duct

Muscle cells—
Oxytocin makes
them contract

Gland cells—
prolactin makes
them secrete

Breastfeeding stimulates the increase of oxytocin and prolactin,
hormones that cause the milk ducts to contract and secrete milk.

◆ WHAT AFFECTS THE CONTENT OF MY BREASTMILK?

Pregnant women usually pay close attention to their diet,
since every food, beverage, and drug they ingest may make its
way to their baby. Fortunately, this is not exactly the case with
breastmilk. Breastmilk is produced from the mammary glands in
your breasts, not directly from the substances you ingest. These
glands draw on the resources available in the form of nutrients
from your diet and from your body's stores of nutrients. If your
diet contains insufficient calories or nutrients to fully sustain
both you and your nursing child, your mammary glands will have
"first shot" at your body's available nutrients to produce highly
nutritious breastmilk, leaving you to rely on whatever is left over.
So a less-than-ideal diet will probably not affect your breastfeeding child, but it may leave *your body* at nutritional risk. (If you
have any concerns that you may not be getting the proper

amount of nutrients, talk to your doctor or nutritionist about improving your diet or the possibility of taking supplements.)

The mammary glands and cells that produce milk also help regulate how much of what you eat and drink actually reaches your baby. Moderate consumption of coffee, tea, caffeinated sodas, and an occasional glass of wine or other alcoholic beverage are fine when you are breastfeeding. However, some babies are more sensitive than others, so keep a close eye on your baby to see how she reacts. It is also reassuring to know that the drugs injected for epidural blocks and other types of regional anesthesia during childbirth do not pass into breastmilk sufficiently to cause long-term harm, though they may make your baby a little sleepy at first. In cases when general anesthesia is used, your anesthesiologist or obstetrician should be informed in advance of your plans to breastfeed.

Most medications are safe to take during breastfeeding, but there are a few—including some nonprescription substances—that may be harmful to the baby. These are not always the same medications that are dangerous for pregnant women to take, so be sure to get approval for all medications from your doctor and your baby's pediatrician.* Excessive alcohol or any kind of recreational drug or medication that has not been approved by your pediatrician should *not* be indulged in, since enough of it could be passed on to your baby and cause serious harm.

AFTER CHILDBIRTH: WHAT HAPPENS NEXT?

As you will find, once you and your baby have settled into a comfortable nursing routine, breastfeeding relies on a wonderful pattern of supply and demand that ensures milk production in just

---

* Since more and more is learned each day about which medications may or may not affect breastfeeding, talk to your doctor about this. Your pediatrician and other healthcare providers may want to refer to the AAP Committee on Drug's recently revised statement, "The Transfer of Drugs and Other Chemicals into Human Milk," in helping to guide you.

the amounts your baby needs at any particular stage of growth. When your baby is especially hungry—in the second to third week of life, during growth spurts when he needs more calories, and so on—he will breastfeed more often, causing your milk production to increase so it can supply extra calories and nutrients. Increased nursing and even more fussiness at these times are normal and temporary. As he grows older and turns to other sources of food, your milk supply will gradually decrease. If at any time you want to increase or decrease the amount of milk you produce, all you need do is adjust the number and length of breastfeeding sessions.

◆ COLOSTRUM: YOUR BABY'S FIRST MEAL

By the time you give birth, your milk-producing cells will have already begun the process of making the thick, yellowish, protein-rich colostrum that will start your baby on the road to good health. Colostrum provides all the nutrients and fluid that your newborn needs in the early days, plus it contains many substances to protect your baby against infections. Its color and thickness are due to the fact that it is higher in these protective factors. (Colostrum is higher in protein, slightly lower in sugar, and significantly lower in fat compared with your more mature breastmilk.) Your body will produce colostrum for several days after delivery until your milk becomes more creamy or white in color and increases in amount—a time that mothers frequently refer to as the milk "coming in."

Your baby will be born with a suckling instinct, though it is stronger in some babies than in others. Since this instinct is at its most intense immediately after birth, it is best to introduce him to the breast within the first hour of life. His suckling at your breast will not only stimulate your breasts to produce more milk, thus beginning the establishment of a reliable milk supply, but it will signal your uterus to contract and decrease the chance of excessive bleeding after delivery. This first feeding will also help him begin to learn how to nurse.

In fact, the initial phase of breastfeeding is a learning process for both mother and baby. Some newborns show little initial interest in nursing. Fortunately, newborns do not need much fluid, and their mothers' breasts contain only small amounts of the very important colostrum. Since the breasts are not yet extremely full of milk, they remain soft and supple after delivery, making it easier for the baby to learn to suckle. It is normal for a baby to lose some weight during his first few days of life. In the days after delivery, your baby's appetite and need for fluids will increase. Between approximately two to five days after birth, the colostrum production will give way to a higher volume of *transitional milk.*

◆ TRANSITIONAL MILK

You may have heard breastfeeding mothers talk about when their milk "came in." They are referring to the onset of production of transitional milk, the creamy breastmilk that immediately follows colostrum and is produced anywhere from about two to five days after birth until ten to fourteen days after birth. Because your breasts will supply a much greater amount of transitional milk than colostrum, your breasts will become larger and firmer during this stage. This new fullness may feel uncomfortable at first and may make it more difficult for your baby to latch on to the breast correctly. With practice, however (and perhaps the help of your baby's pediatrician or lactation specialist), you will help your baby latch on and continued breastfeeding will ease the pressure in your breasts.

As your baby latches on and begins to breastfeed steadily, you may notice a tingly "pins and needles" sensation. This feeling tells you that the milk let-down reflex has begun, causing breastmilk to be pushed out of the milk-producing cells into milk ducts and sinuses so it's available to your baby. The let-down reflex can be stimulated by your baby's suckling, an approaching feeding time, or just the sound of your baby's hungry cry. Once this happens, your milk will flow more plentifully and your baby will enjoy a satisfying feeding. You will hear him swallowing more

This baby is latched on properly and compressing the milk sinuses.

frequently. You may notice milk dripping or spurting from your other breast when let-down occurs.

The combination of sharply increased demand and the resulting increased breastmilk supply may make you feel like you are constantly breastfeeding during this early period. Daytime feedings may be less than two hours apart and last anywhere from ten minutes to close to an hour each. Soon, however, the nursing pattern will stabilize, and feedings will become less frequent. Over time, feedings will continue to change in frequency and length depending on your baby's needs.

◆ **MATURE MILK**

In most women, mature milk begins to appear near the end of the second week after childbirth. Mature milk is produced in as great a volume as transitional milk but is thinner and more watery or even bluish; sometimes it's described as looking like skim milk. Your breasts may appear somewhat softer and smaller than they did during the transitional-milk stage, though they will still be larger than before your pregnancy. These changes in your breasts and in your milk are normal and are designed to provide just what your baby needs for his nutrition, growth, and development.

Much later, after your baby begins to sample other liquids and solid foods, breastfeeding sessions will decrease in frequency. Some mothers and babies choose to continue breastfeeding into the toddler or preschool years. By this time, the overall nutritional contribution of breastfeeding has diminished proportionate to the great variety of other beverages and solids the child is consuming. However, the emotional and immunologic benefits of the nursing relationship continue.

BREASTFEEDING METHODS: WHAT ARE MY ALTERNATIVES?

When most women imagine breastfeeding, they picture themselves nursing breast-to-mouth with their infant cradled in their arms. Certainly this is the most common form of breastfeeding and, as it affords physical contact and an emotional connection for mother and baby, is the most fully satisfying form. However, if you are unable to directly nurse your baby for medical reasons (your baby's premature status, your own serious illness) or practical ones (your temporary absence), alternative methods of giving your child breastmilk are available. In Chapter 9, you will learn how to use a manual or electric breast pump to express milk from your breasts and store it in the refrigerator or freezer for later use. Expressed milk can be fed to any baby whose mother is away at work, at school, shopping, or absent for other reasons. It can be fed to a premature baby with a dropper, spoon, or bottle and to an older baby in a bottle or cup. As your baby gets older, your partner can feed him with your expressed milk to share in the feeding process or let you get some extra sleep. Throughout this book, you will find plenty of ways to provide your baby with breastmilk in one form or another.

The small percentage of mothers who cannot use their own milk to feed their babies may have the option of obtaining other mothers' processed, pasteurized breastmilk that has been donated to milk banks in much the same way that blood is commonly donated. Donated breastmilk does not provide full protection against diseases in the environment, since it must be heat-treated to destroy any potentially dangerous bacteria, viruses, or other infectious particles, but it does provide some of the immune benefits and many of the nutrients that formula does not supply.

A FRIEND IN NEED

Christine, a first-time mother, listened carefully to what her friend Beatrice said about the surprising aspects of breastfeeding. To make sure she was more prepared, she read a book about breastfeeding, talked with members of a breastfeeding support group, and got the name of an available lactation specialist before her baby was born. Once her son, Trevor, was born, Christine was rewarded for her efforts by the confidence with which she was able to initiate a breastfeeding relationship with her son. Each time she witnessed a new change she'd learned about while pregnant—the appearance of colostrum, the increased heaviness of her breasts as her milk volume increased—she congratulated herself on having done her homework so well.

Still, there were surprises. Christine had not realized how tired she would feel at first as she breastfed so frequently, day and night. All new mothers, whether breastfeeding or not, experience this fatigue. Christine soon learned that turning to Beatrice or one of her expert advisers helped fill in the gaps of her newly acquired knowledge. "Nothing beats experience," Beatrice reminded Christine. As you learn all you can about breastfeeding your baby, make a list of resources available to you for specific help or support when needed. Like Christine, you may find during your life as a breastfeeding mother that nothing beats experience and the support of knowledgeable experts and friends.

CHAPTER 3

Getting Ready for Your Baby

"I found that talking to others who were successful at breastfeeding increased my confidence. I guess I felt that if they could learn how to do it, I could too."

—Marjorie, 23, mother of Elaine

Sarah's appointment wasn't until two o'clock, but she was so eager to meet the doctor who might become her baby's pediatrician that she arrived early. As she sat in the waiting room watching other parents play with their children, she wondered: *What will it be like to have a baby? Will I be as happy as these people seem to be? Will my baby be happy with me?*

In one corner of the room, a woman picked up her fussing one-year-old from the play area and settled him into her arms to breastfeed. Sarah opened a parenting magazine and pretended to read but couldn't resist glancing occasionally at the nursing mother. *Now, that's where I really have some questions,* she thought. Early in her pregnancy, Sarah read how important breastmilk is for babies' health and had decided that she wanted to breastfeed her child. She had visited her obstetrician for a breast exam and signed up for a breastfeeding course. Now she was interviewing pediatricians in search of one whose breastfeeding, parenting, and health philosophies were compatible with hers.

Still, Sarah felt unsure about some of the details regarding breastfeeding, as well as childbirth and parenting. *How do you know when they've had enough to eat?* she wondered, glancing at the nursing mother, whose son had fallen asleep in her arms. *Is it okay to let the baby fall asleep like that?* She sighed. *I think I'm going to need some help after this baby is born*, she thought as the receptionist called her name. She stood up, pen and notebook in hand. *Well, at least I'm finding out where to get it.*

Concerned as Sarah felt about her ability to succeed as a breastfeeding mother, she would soon find that she'd done an excellent job preparing for her post-childbirth experience. Visiting your obstetrician for a breast exam, attending breastfeeding classes, and putting together a network of post-childbirth support are all ways to ensure breastfeeding success before your baby is born. Attending ahead of time to practical issues—such as health-insurance coverage, child-care issues, and your plan for breastfeeding at the workplace—can also make it easier to focus on your baby after the birth. In this chapter, you will find a number of ways to get ready for your baby, inform yourself as fully as possible about how breastfeeding works, and put together an optimal "support team" to help you with any questions that come up later. The more you lay the groundwork now, the more you and your baby will benefit.

CAN I BREASTFEED?
PREPARING YOUR BODY FOR NURSING

Breastfeeding is a natural process that requires no special physical preparation for most women. However, you should discuss your plans to breastfeed with your obstetrician/gynecologist and have him examine your breasts as early as possible in your pregnancy and again during the third trimester. Tell him about any breastfeeding or early weaning problems you've had with previous children, or of any breast biopsies, breast enhancement, reduction, or other breast surgery you've experienced. Also, make sure he knows of any chronic medical problems or illnesses you have. Chances are excellent that he will tell you he foresees no trouble in your ability to produce enough milk for your baby, even if you have experienced one or more of these situations. (See Chapter 5 for more information about the effects of breast surgery on nursing.) However, if you have had problems before or the condition of your breasts suggest special challenges ahead, being aware of these potential hindrances can make all the difference in your ability to successfully breastfeed.

As discussed in Chapter 2, small breast size does not predict an insufficient milk supply for the baby, but women whose breasts do not enlarge at least somewhat during pregnancy (regardless of their pre-pregnancy breast size) may experience difficulty in producing sufficient milk. This is not the case for every mother whose breasts remain relatively unchanged, but it is a "caution" sign your obstetrician should note on your prenatal record and communicate to your pediatrician, lactation specialist, and other medical personnel. This helps ensure that your baby's milk intake will be monitored carefully to see that she is getting enough nourishment.

Your obstetrician should note other variations in breast size or shape. Large breasts can make it awkward to hold the baby in a correct position to nurse, or make it hard for the baby to latch on to the breast. Breasts of markedly unequal size may lead to a normal supply of milk in one breast but little milk produced by the other. Tubular or elongated breasts sometimes contain an insufficient number of milk glands; breastfeeding in these cases should be closely monitored to be sure enough milk is being produced. Again, please understand that none of these characteristics means that you will be unable to breastfeed successfully. They simply mean that your health-care professionals should pay close attention to early breastfeeding, make sure everything is proceeding smoothly, and offer you solutions to any problems that arise.

◆ INVERTED OR FLAT NIPPLES

One breast characteristic you should certainly point out to your obstetrician and pediatrician is inverted or flat nipples. In-

A normally protruding—or everted—nipple becomes erect when you press the areola between two fingers.

verted nipples retract inward toward the breast instead of protruding out when the areola is gently squeezed. Flat nipples neither retract nor protrude, but remain more or less flat. When not compressed, some inverted nipples appear normal. Others contain a small dimple or may have a clear indentation at all times. You can "test" your own nipples by gently squeezing the areola about one to two inches behind the nipple. If your nipples draw inward or remain flat, tell your obstetrician and pediatrician.

Inverted nipples, and to a lesser extent flat nipples, can create a problem during breastfeeding by making it more difficult for the baby to properly latch on to the breast. In some cases, inverted nipples may actually impede the flow of milk. They are also more prone to injury of the nipple surface. Fortunately, inverted and flat nipples sometimes become sufficiently everted, or normally protruding, on their own during pregnancy so by the

Inverted nipples retract toward the breast when pressure is applied to the areola.

time the baby is born, breastfeeding can proceed without prob-lems. If not, this characteristic should not prevent most women from successfully breastfeeding their children; solutions to this relatively common problem are in Chapter 4.

Some methods used in the past to correct inverted nipples during pregnancy may actually reduce breastfeeding success and are no longer routinely recommended. These include the use of breast shells—plastic cups with a hole in the center that are pressed against the breasts, leaving the nipples exposed. (Breast shells may be helpful after childbirth, although their benefit has not been proved in studies. See Chapter 4.) Manual exercises to encourage the nipples to protrude, called nipple rolling, have no effect. Experts now agree that it is best to wait until after child-birth to address inverted nipples—but your medical support team should certainly be informed about your situation.

Flat nipples neither retract nor protrude, remaining more or less flat.

Pierced Nipples

In most cases, pierced nipples do not interfere with breastfeeding, though any rings or studs should be removed prior to a breast-feeding session to prevent choking. If your piercing became infected at the time of the piercing or later, inform your doctor. Such infection, as well as any scarring that may have occurred, can make nursing more difficult. While breastfeeding, some of your breast-milk may leak through the pierced hole. This is usually not a problem, but if you have any questions be sure to ask your pediatrician or a lactation specialist to check that your baby is nursing well.

◆ CHANGES IN YOUR BREASTS

As was noted in the previous chapter, physical changes in your breasts will occur as your pregnancy continues and your body prepares for nursing. Your breasts will grow larger and may begin to secrete colostrum. These small secretions can leave yellow stains on your clothing. In rare cases, the stains may be rust-colored or brown. This means they contain some blood—also usually a result of normal breast development—but do mention this to your obstetrician.

Many women experience a new tenderness in their nipples. This is also a normal aspect of pregnancy, though sometimes it can be exacerbated by a dry climate or rough-textured clothing worn next to the skin. While experts used to encourage expectant mothers to use creams, lotions, "toughening-up" exercises, and other techniques to decrease nipple sensitivity and prepare for nursing, it is now believed that nature offers the best preparation. In fact, your body secretes a lubricating and cleansing substance through small, raised areas on the areolae called Montgomery's glands. Usually, this is all that's needed to prevent undue dryness. If you find that your nipples continue to feel extremely sensitive, dry, and flaky as childbirth approaches, try keeping them uncovered for an hour or more a day. If that doesn't work, apply a small amount of medical-grade lanolin, labeled as purified (available at most pharmacies or through a lactation specialist).

◆ MEDICATION

At the time of your breast exam or as soon as possible after you have learned that you are pregnant, inform your obstetrician about any medications you are currently taking or know you will be taking after childbirth. She will be able to tell you if your medication is safe and may be able to provide you with a safe substitute if it is not. If you are told that you cannot breastfeed while taking the drug, get a second opinion. (Many professionals are unsure about issues of drugs in breastmilk and prefer to err on the side of caution.) It is important to clear up any confusion long before your due date approaches, since the hospital staff may be uncomfortable with your breastfeeding if they are unfamiliar with the use of your medication during lactation.

Can I Breastfeed Too?

PREPARING FOR YOUR ADOPTED BABY

If you are adopting a newborn or older baby in the near future, you may know of adoptive mothers who breastfed their children and wonder whether you might do the same.

You will find more detailed information about adoptive breastfeeding in Chapter 5. In the meantime, if you are considering this, talk with your doctor and pediatrician, as well as a lactation specialist or your local La Leche League representative. They can help you assess your specific situation and your future baby's needs, instruct you on how to stimulate milk production, supplement feedings with donated breastmilk or formula, and even put you in touch with other adoptive mothers who have successfully breastfed. Since induced lactation works best with a newborn or younger baby, it's best to research this issue sooner rather than later. Ideally, you will want to begin inducing lactation two weeks to one month before your baby arrives.

WHAT ELSE DO I NEED TO KNOW?
GATHERING INFORMATION ABOUT
BREASTFEEDING

"When I was pregnant, I went after the facts of parenting like a reporter going after a story," said Anthea, mother of Ginny. "I did as much research as possible ahead of time, because I knew that after the baby was born I would want to focus on her. Once I started breastfeeding Ginny, new questions came up that I hadn't thought of during the pregnancy. But at least I started out with a firm base of knowledge and a list of good professionals who could help me."

You and your partner will benefit greatly by taking time before your baby's birth to learn all you can about the mechanics of breastfeeding. Books such as this one can answer many of your questions. (And if you read all the way through you'll know where to find specific information once you have the baby.) The fact is, though, that with breastfeeding nothing beats personal guidance from an expert. We recommend, if possible, taking a breastfeeding course that lasts for several sessions.

Your obstetrician or pediatrician may be able to refer you to a good breastfeeding course in your area. Hospitals frequently provide such courses and may offer private consultations with a lactation specialist as well. Another option is to attend meetings offered by La Leche League International, a nonprofit organization with chapters in nearly every American city. La Leche League, founded in the 1950s by a group of Chicago mothers who saw a need for mother-to-mother support in breastfeeding, provides nursing women with individual help through breastfeeding meetings, in-person and telephone counseling, informative publications, information via the Internet, and even special equipment when necessary. Many couples have expressed their enthusiasm that all La Leche League counselors—including those who conduct instructional meetings—are experienced mothers who have themselves breastfed. They understand exactly what new mothers are going through and also can talk about other parenting issues. Attending the meetings before you give birth will help you familiarize yourself with what other services your local group offers and decide whether this approach suits your personal philosophy and style. (See "Breastfeeding Resources" contact information.)

Government initiatives such as the WIC program (the Special Supplemental Nutrition Program for Women, Infants, and Children) also offer breastfeeding courses or counseling. The WIC program, operated by the U.S. Department of Agriculture in partnership with state and local health departments, provides other services as well—including one-on-one prenatal breastfeeding education, nutrition information, health-care referrals, postpartum follow-up and counseling, peer support programs, and extra food—to families whose income is below a certain level. The maximum allowable income changes from year to year but is not as low as might be expected. About sixty percent of infants born in 1998 were eligible to receive WIC's services, and almost three-fourths did so. To find out whether you qualify, call your local or state health department, listed in your local phone book, or see "Breastfeeding Resources."

What a Course Can't Cover

Breastfeeding courses cover a wide array of situations that new parents experience, but if your particular circumstances require additional help you may need to dig further for information. Parents expecting twins or greater multiples, for example, should contact the local chapter of their National Organization of Mothers of Twins club (see "Breastfeeding Resources") for advice on how to breastfeed multiples, what (if any) special equipment you may need, and what kind of extra help you may want to secure for your return home after birth. Since there is a greater chance that your babies may be born prematurely, you should also find out how to provide your infants with breastmilk if they are unable to nurse at first. (See Chapter 5.) If you know your baby will be born with a birth defect, such as a cleft palate, heart defect, or other medical problem that may affect her ability to nurse, dedicate some time now to researching your child's condition and contacting appropriate support groups (see "Breastfeeding Resources").

If you suffer from a medical problem such as chronic depression, anxiety disorder, hepatitis, TB, or any infectious disease that may prevent you from nursing, discuss the issue as soon as possible with your pediatrician, obstetrician, and the doctor who is treating you for the illness. Most medical conditions are compatible with breastfeeding, but you will want to be sure.

All parents who expect to confront a special situation regarding breastfeeding should discuss the issue with their obstetrician and their child's pediatrician before the birth. Your doctor can refer you to a lactation specialist (or one may be available at the hospital where you will give birth) who can talk with you about how to successfully breastfeed. Your La Leche League contact can also provide you with valuable advice, support, and references in all of these areas and can in most cases put you in touch with other mothers who have breastfed successfully under similar circumstances.

Attending breastfeeding classes makes at least as much sense as partaking in a more traditional childbirth course, since you will spend more time breastfeeding than you will giving birth. Breastfeeding instruction is even more important now that your postpartum hospital stay can be as short as twenty-four hours. By attending a class and preparing in other ways, you can ensure that you will be reasonably well prepared long *before* you arrive at the hospital. Be sure to ask anyone else who expects to help you begin breastfeeding to attend these classes as well, to learn how best to support you and your baby and to explore their role as a nonbreastfeeding caregiver.

WHO WILL BE THERE IF I NEED HELP? CREATING A NETWORK OF POSTPARTUM SUPPORT

In traditional societies, new mothers have always relied on other, experienced women to help them with the most common questions and concerns regarding breastfeeding. Today, in this country, we also have the more knowledgeable assistance of such trained experts as pediatricians, hospital nurses, lactation specialists, and La Leche League volunteers. Since breastfeeding is a learned skill—not an instinctive process—such advice is always helpful. If you have trouble establishing a nursing pattern after childbirth, you may find it indispensable.

◆ THE RIGHT HOSPITAL

To ensure a successful start for breastfeeding, choose a breastfeeding-friendly location in which to give birth—a place where mothers are encouraged to stay with their newborns around the clock (called "rooming in") and babies are not offered pacifiers or supplemental feedings that will interfere with their ability to nurse. In recent years many hospitals have become more active in this area as the demand for breastfeeding has increased, but be sure to check.

Tour the hospitals that are available to you and ask your tour guide what the facility's maternity policies are. Does this hospital officially encourage breastfeeding on demand, and are all health staff instructed to implement and support this policy? Are mothers and babies kept together immediately after birth and helped to initiate breastfeeding within the first hour? Are supplemental feedings given only for medical reasons or if the mother has requested otherwise? Are babies allowed to stay in the mother's room full-time? Ask whether the hospital or birthing center maintains one or more lactation specialists on staff and whether the regular nursing staff both supports breastfeeding and spends time helping new mothers learn to nurse. Finally, find out whether they routinely refer new mothers to breastfeeding support groups in the area and other sources of postpartum help. Some hospitals and birthing centers in the United States have been certified as Baby Friendly Hospitals, which means that the hospital has complied with a specified ten-step process of training, education, and support to provide breastfeeding mothers and babies with the best start in breastfeeding. (The Baby Friendly Hospital Initiative, developed internationally by UNICEF, the World Health Organization, and other organizations such as Wellstart International, is administered in the United States by Baby Friendly USA.)

Your choice of a hospital or birthing center may be limited by geographic location, insurance or HMO coverage, and doctor–hospital affiliations. Inspecting busy hospitals can sometimes be intimidating. Keep in mind, however, that childbirth is a competitive market in this country and your business is wanted. Choose a facility that will help you begin your life with your baby in the way you know is best.

◆ THE RIGHT PEDIATRICIAN

Another invaluable source of breastfeeding support in the period immediately following childbirth is your child's pediatrician. Since this medical professional may need to make decisions regarding feedings immediately after childbirth, when you may or may not be able to participate depending on your medical condition, it is important to choose the most appropriate person ahead of time and communicate your plans for breastfeeding.

The best way to create a "shortlist" of potential pediatricians is to solicit recommendations from friends with babies or young children, your obstetrician, your hospital or birthing center, and the volunteers at your local La Leche League. Once you've collected several names, interview each candidate, selecting one who inspires your confidence and with whom you feel a certain amount of personal affinity. Be sure he or she is knowledgeable and supportive of breastfeeding practices, aware of any potential problems you have discovered, and willing to support your efforts to nurse from the beginning. You might want to ask the pediatrician the following questions—but be sure to customize this list to suit your own needs.

- What percentage of the infants in your practice are breast-fed?
- How soon after birth do you recommend that a mother begin breastfeeding?
- What is your opinion regarding rooming-in for mother and baby?
- How long do you typically recommend exclusive breastfeeding?
- About how long do most of the mothers in your practice breastfeed?
- How will I be able to tell if my breastfed baby is getting enough milk and growing properly?
- Is there an age at which you recommend weaning?
- What are your views on mothers of babies returning to work?

Don't hesitate to ask for time just to talk. Pediatricians understand that it's important for parents to find an appropriate caregiver for their child. Few patient–doctor matches are absolutely perfect, but you should feel a certain amount of personal ease with your child's doctor. In some situations, you may choose a family physician to care for your child, in which case the same selection process would apply.

◆ MORE BREASTFEEDING SUPPORT

You can secure support from professionals trained specifically in breastfeeding practices before you have your baby as well. These advisers—volunteer breastfeeding consultants, baby nurses, doulas (women who care for the mother during labor, delivery, and after childbirth so she can focus on her baby), and lactation specialists—may be recommended by your obstetrician, made available by your hospital or birthing center, or may even be suggested by other mothers who have benefited from their services.

Lactation specialists come from a variety of backgrounds. Many are nurses with special expertise in mother–baby care. Others are certified IBCLCs (International Board Certified Lactation Consultants) who have completed course work, clinical practice hours, and passed a standardized exam that covers infant feeding, breast anatomy, milk production, management of breastfeeding complications, and stages of infant development. Unlike a nurse or physician, the IBCLC designation alone does not mean a person is licensed by the state to practice in the capacity of a health-care professional, but most IBCLCs do have a great deal of experience working with breastfeeding mothers. It's a good idea to interview a potential lactation specialist before the birth, if possible, to discuss such issues as training, number of nursing mothers assisted, fee structures, references, and the possibility and frequency of postpartum visits to your home or at her office. You might also inquire about backup arrangements in case she is unavailable.

◆ FAMILY SUPPORT

Ideally, by your due date you will have formed relationships with a pediatrician, members of your local La Leche League, and/or WIC office, and perhaps a doula, baby nurse, or lactation specialist. Now is also the time to assemble the family members and friends whom you expect to support you in this new venture. Talk with your baby's father about how he can make it possible for you to focus on the baby during the first vital weeks of breastfeeding. (See Chapter 11 for ideas about this.) Talk with your older children, if you have any, in a matter-of-fact way about how you will breastfeed this baby and what they might do to help. (More information about older siblings is also available in Chapter 6.) Welcome offers from other family members to help as long as they understand and support your determination to breastfeed. Well-meaning friends and loved ones believe they are helping when they offer to give the baby a bottle or ignore the baby's demands for a feeding to "let you get some rest." But you will not want or need anyone, no matter how close, to discourage you from getting breastfeeding off to a good start. If you feel this may happen, provide your helper with other activities (washing dishes, doing laundry, changing the baby's diaper, playing with her) that can help you get some rest or ask her to visit a couple of months after the birth, when your nursing routine has been established.

IS THE PAPERWORK DONE?

While you are pregnant, it's important to take care of any practical chores relating to breastfeeding. Before you leave work on maternity leave, for example, you will want to talk with your employer and determine how you can provide breastmilk for your baby after your return. In Chapter 10, you will find information on how to secure a private space and regular breaks for expressing breastmilk on the job, and you'll learn how to store your breastmilk so your child's caregiver can feed it to him in a bottle or cup. By reviewing this information before the birth, you can make a plan that best suits your work and home situations. It's best to put your agreement in writing with your employer before you leave to have your baby so you'll feel more confident about your return to work and your employer will be reassured that you do intend to return.

While you are thinking about your return to work, you may also give some thought to how well your baby's caregiver or child-care center will follow the practices and instructions you set for feeding your baby. (This issue is discussed at greater length in Chapter 9.) If you are currently in the process of choosing a caregiver or child-care program, you will need to discuss your breastfeeding plans in the interview or conversation. Your baby's caregivers must be comfortable with the idea of handling bottles filled with your breastmilk, for example, and must agree to follow your directions regarding formula supplements, whether and when to introduce solid foods, and so on. Bring up the relevant issues *during your first talks* with a potential caregiver, rather than waiting until the weeks or days before you return to your job.

Since you may require the services of a lactation specialist or need to rent a breast pump or other breastfeeding equipment after your baby is born, review your health-insurance policy or HMO agreement now to see if it covers such services. If these costs will not be reimbursed, consider budgeting for what you might need or talk to your plan administrator about getting breastfeeding services covered. Many insurance companies are now aware of the many health benefits and the decreased health-care costs associated with breastfeeding and are interested in investing in services that support breastfeeding. Be sure you have identified any community resources that will provide you with breastfeeding help should the need arise.

One final bit of paperwork involves your plan for exclusively breastfeeding your baby while still at the hospital. While most hospital policies have made progress toward supporting exclusive breastfeeding, ask your obstetrician to include specific instruction in your birthing plan regarding your desire to avoid feeding supplements for your baby and to keep him with you in your room. Studies have shown that newborns adjust most easily to breastfeeding when they are not provided with alternatives such as formula, water, or even pacifiers. Also inform your husband, partner, or other birthing coach about your desire to breastfeed soon after childbirth, and remind your obstetrician and obstetrical nurses about this, if possible, early in your labor.

WHAT DO I NEED TO BREASTFEED?
OPTIONAL AIDS TO MAKE
NURSING EASIER

Throughout most of human history, mothers have successfully breastfed their babies without the help of nursing pillows, breast pads, or even rocking chairs. Our bodies, and our children's bodies, are well-designed to make nursing a simple and rewarding process. Still, some supplies can make life as a nursing mother easier, if they fit into your budget. (Nursing equipment also makes wonderful baby gifts.)

A well-made nursing bra that comfortably supports your enlarged breasts can be useful. It is difficult to predict what size nursing bra you will need, but take your best guess and purchase at least one or two while pregnant to have for the hospital. After childbirth you can be fitted for one, which should never be tight or constricting. Nursing bras have front flaps that can be detached with one hand (while the other is supporting the baby) and pulled open for nursing. Outer clothing designed for nursing provides openings for the baby and is a

Nursing bras provide proper support and have front flaps that can be detached with one hand.

practical idea for mothers concerned about nursing discreetly in public. Both nursing bras and clothing are available at maternity shops, in mother–child clothing catalogs, and at many department stores. Of course, shirts that can easily be lifted up and blouses that unbutton from the bottom up also work quite well.

Disposable or washable breast pads, which can be slipped inside the bra cup to absorb any milk that leaks out between feedings, are useful for women

Shirts that can be lifted with one hand make nursing easier.

whose breasts leak a great deal or who sometimes find themselves away from their babies at a regular feeding time. Avoid pads with plastic liners that impede the flow of air around the nipples and hold the moisture in, which can irritate the nipples. Breast pads can be purchased at most pharmacies and grocery stores— though a folded piece of absorbent cloth works almost as well.

While not necessary for successful breastfeeding, equipment to help you hold, cuddle, and soothe your baby can be a welcome addition to a nursery. Some mothers find that a custom-made nursing pillow, designed to help you position your baby properly and hold her for an entire feeding without tiring your arms, is easier than trying to arrange ordinary pillows or cushions. (Nursing pillows come in various shapes and sizes, so you may want to try out several before choosing one that suits you.) A footstool raises the level of your lap, bringing your baby closer to your breast. It also helps keep your back straight, which may make you more comfortable. Some new mothers en-

Packing Your Bag

WHAT TO TAKE TO THE HOSPITAL

While the average hospital stay for a new mother and baby has decreased significantly over recent years, there's still no way to predict whether you will be away from home for a day or for a week. So it's a good idea to pack some breastfeeding supplies along with your toiletry bag and a list of friends and relatives to call.

The nursing bras you bought during your pregnancy are definite items to put into the suitcase. While you might not wear them during your hospital stay, you could check the fit after childbirth or practice unhooking the front flap one-handed before you nurse. A nightgown with slits at the breasts for easy, discreet nursing is also helpful when you expect visitors outside your immediate family, though with practice you will soon find it easy to breastfeed with reasonable modesty even with non-nursing clothes. Some women pack breast pads, though these are rarely necessary in the early days, when the amount of colostrum or milk being produced is small and leaking is uncommon. Nursing pillows to support the baby while breastfeeding and medical-grade lanolin to soothe tender nipples may not be necessary this early in the process—but if it reassures you to know they'll be nearby, by all means bring them. And pack this book as well; at two in the morning, when your partner is asleep and the lactation specialist is not available, you may find answers to your most urgent questions here.

joy a rocking chair or glider to use in the baby's room in antic-ipation of those precious moments when a nursing session blends into sleep.

Other pieces of optional equipment include a baby sling or carrier that frees your hands while keeping your baby close enough to nurse, and a bassinet for keeping your sleeping infant beside your bed. You can find these items in most baby-supply stores and baby-equipment catalogs. Please remember, however, that special equipment and furnishings are all "extras." All you really need to nurse successfully are your breasts and a hungry baby.

THE BIG DAY

Why do so many babies decide to enter the world in the early hours of the morning? All the way to the hospital, Sarah kept her eyes on the pink horizon where the sun would soon appear, while her husband, Bob, drove the car. Soon they arrived at the hospital entrance, literally on the threshold of parenthood. *By this time tomorrow I'll have my baby in my arms*, Sarah thought as her husband guided her toward the admissions desk. Fortunately, she had spent time preparing for this moment and the many days and months to follow. She'd attended a breastfeeding class, knew whom to call if and when questions arose, and was aware that her hospital supported a doula being present during labor and deliv-ery to provide constant support. Her best friend from college, an experienced breastfeeding mother, had promised to help for a week or so as well. And Sarah knew that the wonderful pediatri-cian she'd found would provide excellent care for the baby. Everything was in place—and that was reassuring, because this baby was giving every sign that he was ready to make an appear-ance *right now*.

Now is the time for you, too, to prepare the best possible en-vironment for your baby's arrival. Breastfeeding is a natural process, but it always begins more easily with a little help from professionals, relatives, and friends. For many new mothers, the first few weeks after childbirth pass in an exciting blur. Use the time you have now to give the future you—you as a breastfeeding mother—a helping hand.

CHAPTER 4

The First Feedings

*"I knew that breastfeeding was the best for my child as the
natural transition from pregnancy to parenting. Most
important, it was something that only I could give my child.
Anybody can bottle-feed, but breastfeeding was
something only I could do for him."*

—Ellen, 40, mother of Frank

"It's a boy!" Tired as Teresa was after twelve hours of labor, the
obstetrician's words filled her with euphoria. *My baby's here!* she
told herself, hardly able to believe it as her newborn was placed
on her stomach. Teresa, a single mother, had brought her best
friend, Linda, along to act as birthing coach. Linda stepped back
as the nurse dried the baby's head with a towel. "Hello, little
baby," Teresa murmured. "Hello, Gabriel."

Baby Gabriel, alert and clearly astonished by his new surroundings, soon started to inch up toward Teresa's breast. "Hey,
what's he doing?" Teresa said, surprised.

"He wants to nurse," Linda said. "Remember? They said in the
breastfeeding class that he might do that. Anyway, you're sup-
posed to try to nurse in the first hour."

As Gabriel worked his way up her chest, Teresa cradled her
baby to her breast. Gabriel's look of amazement as he tasted the
nipple made Teresa laugh. He started to latch on but then pulled
back and looked around. "Oops, he stopped," Teresa said, disappointed but not surprised. Her breastfeeding instructor had said
that this kind of hesitation happens sometimes.

Teresa was so intent on this first interaction with her newborn that she hardly noticed the bustle of activity surrounding her. Medical personnel seemed to fill the room, filling out forms, moving equipment, and straightening up the birthing area. "Excuse me," Linda said to one of the nurses. "Teresa's planning to breastfeed. She wanted to make sure her baby isn't given any formula or pacifiers, okay?"

"Right." The nurse checked the orders. "That's our hospital policy for breastfed babies. We encourage rooming in so you will be able to breastfeed your baby on demand. Is that what you're planning?"

"Uh-huh." Teresa smiled down at Gabriel. Tentatively, she moved him toward her breast again. This time Gabriel focused intently on the nipple. His mouth opened wide and, as Teresa cradled him, he latched on fully and started to suckle. "Look, he's doing it!" Teresa said excitedly to Linda.

FIRST ENCOUNTER

The minutes following childbirth are typically an exciting, confusing, and emotionally chaotic time for everyone involved. As you recover from your physical ordeal, you may feel overwhelmed by an enormous number of new feelings, hopes, and uncertainties. Of course, this is also a time when you want the professional treatment of your newborn to proceed according to your wishes. Ideally, you will have informed your obstetrician and pediatrician ahead of time of your desire to breastfeed, as recommended in Chapter 3. Your partner or birthing coach should remind your pediatrician and obstetrical nurses that you do not want your baby to be given water, a pacifier, or supplemental feedings without a valid medical reason.

You will want to breastfeed within an hour of giving birth to take advantage of your baby's suckling instinct when your baby is awake and alert. Immediate breastfeeding also starts the process of establishing your future milk supply and helps your uterus contract and return to its pre-pregnancy state, which decreases the chance of excessive bleeding after delivery. Breastfeeding immediately is possible with most healthy births, when a baby needs little medical care beyond drying off and keeping warm by being placed skin-to-skin against your naked abdomen or chest. Offering your breast to your infant at this time will help her take advantage of her natural instincts to get breastfeeding off to a great start.

This is not to say that your newborn will instantly know what to do. Some mothers find that their babies do not actively suckle during the first few attempts—but instead simply snuggle contentedly against the breast, tentatively lick the nipple, or attach to the breast and suckle briefly but then stop and look around. Many others find that their babies latch on right away and suckle as if they've been doing it for months. (Most babies suck on their fingers or arms in the uterus.) Whether or not your infant actually breast-

Breastfeeding immediately after birth helps establish your milk supply and encourages your baby's natural instinct to nurse.

feeds productively at this time is not critical. Rather, this is a time for the two of you to start to get to know each other, for her to be introduced to the breast, and for her to begin to associate the sight, smell, and feel of your breasts with the quenching of her hunger.

This first feeding is important for you, too, in that it represents your first step in establishing a breastfeeding relationship. No matter how well you have prepared ahead of time, your first real breastfeeding experience may feel a little strange. Your baby's tongue on your nipple or her firm grip on your breast may feel different than you'd imagined, or you may find that you are unsure whether you are holding her correctly or whether she's truly latched on. You may perceive help from nurses as intrusive or feel self-conscious trying to breastfeed in a room full of strangers. All of these feelings are normal for a new mother. As in any partnership, you and your newborn will have to learn and adjust to each other's style; as with any physical skill, full mastery will come with practice. For now it's best to relax, enjoy this moment, and wait until you've both had some rest before worrying about perfecting your technique.

There are some situations in which immediate breastfeeding is not possible or advisable. If your baby is premature, ill, in fragile condition, or if you are still struggling to recover from medication given for a cesarean section or any other type of sedation, you may need to postpone nursing. (For special issues such as cesarean sections, premature birth, and illness, see Chapter 5.) If this is the case, there is still plenty of time to introduce yourselves to each other. Then focus on getting the immediate help you and your baby need so that breastfeeding can go more smoothly at the next feeding.

GETTING TO KNOW YOU: EARLY FEEDINGS

"Those first hours after I had Debbie were all just a blur," reports Judith, a new mother in her early thirties. "I don't remember

A Great Beginning

EARLY BREASTFEEDING BASICS

- Initiate breastfeeding within an hour of birth.

- Request that your baby not be fed any formula, water, or sugar water without a medical reason. Water and sugar water are generally not needed. Do not allow your newborn to be given a pacifier. Ask your obstetrician or pediatrician to write an order to this effect if needed.

- Keep your newborn with you day and night.

- Breastfeed on demand, as soon as your baby shows hunger cues such as increased alertness or activity, smacking her lips, making suckling motions, or rooting (moving her head around in search of your breast). Don't wait until your baby begins to cry, which is a late sign of hunger. Feed for as long as your baby desires, until she detaches spontaneously from each breast.

- Shortly after delivery, and again prior to discharge, have a lactation specialist or nurse experienced in breastfeeding monitor your nursing technique to be sure everything is going well. Request a follow-up evaluation with your pediatrician within forty-eight to seventy-two hours after leaving the hospital (or by the time your baby is three to five days old).

- If you must be separated from your baby and cannot breastfeed directly, express your milk to be given to your baby. (Ask a nurse or lactation specialist for help expressing milk.)

when I fell asleep, who brought Debbie into the room with me, or how long she was there before I woke up. All I know is, she was there when I opened my eyes, and the first thing I wanted to do when my husband brought her to me was get another look at her face and then practice feeding her."

It is exciting, finally making the physical connection with the baby you've been contemplating for so many months. While most mothers and newborns prefer to rest for a few hours following an initial feeding, the time to practice nursing will soon follow. In order to avoid problems later, it is important to begin mastering the basics: how to position yourself, how to hold your baby, and how to make sure she's properly latched on. By practicing correct breastfeeding technique while you're still in the hospital and have immediate access to expert help and support, you can get your baby off to the best possible start.

◆ POSITIONS FOR BREASTFEEDING

Once you and your baby have become old hands at breastfeeding, you'll be able to nurse while talking on the phone, reading a book, supervising your other children, or walking around. For now, though, it's best to start with as few distractions as possible. Most new mothers first try breastfeeding sitting up in a hospital bed, with the baby supported by a pillow in their lap and cradled in their arms. If you choose this position, elevate the head of the bed as much as possible and place pillows behind you until your back is comfortable. Place your baby on a pillow on your lap (this is an especially good idea if you've had a cesarean section, or "C-section") so his head is level with your breast. You might put pillows at your sides to rest your arms so they won't tire mid-feeding. At home, you may find an armchair helpful. If you breastfeed while sitting in a chair, be sure it offers sturdy back and arm support and is not too low or high. A pillow or two tucked behind your back can make nursing in a chair more comfortable, as can a low footstool to support your legs.

Whether you are sitting up in bed or have settled into an armchair, keep your back straight but relaxed as you offer your baby the breast. Your baby may find it more difficult to latch on properly if you are leaning forward or back, since this changes the angle at which he receives the breast; your back may soon feel the strain of this as well. If your breasts are large, you might need to place a rolled-up towel or receiving blanket beneath your breast to keep your baby's mouth at a straight-on angle with the nipple, in addition to supporting the breast with your hand.

Once you are correctly positioned, you can hold your baby in a number of ways. As you practice breastfeeding before leaving the hospital, try several positions (for both your baby and yourself) and ask your nurse or lactation specialist to check your technique. Using more than one position can help prevent nipple soreness and clogging of milk ducts, since different positions drain different areas of the breast more effectively. (For information on clogged milk ducts, see Chapter 8.) Some positions also work better than others in certain circumstances; for example, the reclining position is lovely when you're half-asleep.

The cradle hold is the traditional breastfeeding position.

◆ **THE CRADLE HOLD**

The traditional position is called the *cradle hold* or *Madonna hold*. To do this, support your baby on the arm that's on the same side as the breast you intend to use. Holding your upper arm close to your body, rest your baby's head on the crook of your elbow, support his back with your forearm, and cup his bottom or upper thigh with your hand. His arm may be positioned around your body or tucked slightly under his body to keep it out of the way. Once he's properly supported, rotate your forearm so his entire body turns toward you. His pelvis should be up against your abdomen, his chest against your chest, and his mouth lined up with your nipple. You can now bring your baby's mouth to the nipple (rather than the nipple to his mouth) without making him turn his head to the side. It is important for your baby's head to be aligned with the rest of his body instead of turned off to the side.

◆ **THE CROSSOVER HOLD**

A variation on the cradle hold, the *crossover hold* or *cross-cradle hold* involves the same positioning except you support your baby

The cross-cradle hold is a good position for a baby who has difficulty latching on.

on the arm opposite the breast being used. In this position, your hand supports your baby's neck and upper back, rather than his bottom, and his bottom rests either in the crook of your arm or on the pillow on your lap. Again, rotate your baby's body so it faces you and his mouth is lined up with your nipple. This is a good position for a baby who has difficulty latching on, because you can more easily move his head into a better position by holding the back of his neck between your thumb and fingers.

◆ THE CLUTCH HOLD

Many breastfeeding women find that the *clutch hold*, also known as the *football hold*, is an easier position to maintain, particularly for those who have given birth by cesarean delivery, because it keeps the baby's weight off the abdominal incision. The

The clutch or football hold is an easy position to maintain and is particularly helpful if you've had a cesarean delivery because it keeps the baby's weight off the incision.

clutch hold may also be useful for mothers of twins since one baby can nurse on each side, and for women with large breasts or flat nipples since the mother can see both her nipple and her baby's mouth and can easily control the baby's head. In a clutch hold, your baby is held similar to how you would hold a handbag clutched under your arm or a football clutched close to your body. To feed your baby in this position, place him beside you—on the side of the breast you will use—with his head near your breast. Tuck his body up against your side, under your arm. Your forearm should support his upper back, and your hand and fingers should support his shoulders, neck, and head. His legs will stretch out straight behind you or, if you are in a chair, you can rest his bottom against the back of the chair and angle his legs straight up. Finally, placing a pillow under your elbow for support, keep your baby's head level with your breast.

◆ RECLINING

You may find that feeding your baby in a *reclining* position, rather than sitting, allows for some welcome relaxation. Nursing lying down helps particularly if you have had a cesarean delivery or otherwise feel tired or unwell in the days following childbirth. To do this, lie on your side with one or more pillows behind your back and under your head for support. (A pillow placed between your knees may make you more comfortable.) Keep your back and hips in as straight a line as possible. Hold your baby closely on his side so he faces you with his mouth even with your nipple and your lower arm around him. Support your breast with your other hand while guiding your baby closer with the arm supporting him.

An advantage of the reclining position is you don't have to get up to reposition your baby on your other breast. Simply place a pillow under him to elevate him until he's parallel with your upper breast and lean over further to bring the upper breast to him. Or, if you prefer, hug him to your chest, roll over to your other side, and reposition him. You can even support your baby by placing a pillow behind his back, thus giving your lower arm a rest.

Feeding your baby in a reclining position lets you relax if you've
had a cesarean delivery or feel tired in the days following childbirth.

◆ ENSURING PROPER LATCH-ON

In any of the nursing positions described above, when the
baby is well-aligned you should be able to draw a straight line
that connects the baby's ear, shoulder, and hip on either side of
the baby's body.

Once you and your baby are in proper position, the next step
is to guide him toward the breast so that he can latch on properly
and nurse. In most cases (other than in the reclining position), it
will be necessary to support your breast, at least in the early days
of breastfeeding, in order for your baby to attach properly. This is
especially true as milk production increases your breasts' size and
weight. Using your free hand, place four fingers under your breast
and your thumb on top to present the nipple to your baby. (Your
lactation specialist or nurse may refer to this as a *C-hold*, since your
hand makes the shape of a letter C.) Make sure your fingers are

Using a C-hold, tickle your baby's lower lip with your nipple to stimulate his rooting reflex.

well behind the areola (the darker-colored area around the nipple) so it doesn't get in the way of your baby's latching on to the breast.

With the breast supported, tickle your baby's lower lip with your nipple. This causes him to open his mouth. (If his mouth stays closed, tickle his lip again, press gently down on his chin with your index finger, and open your own mouth, too, since he might imitate you.) When he opens wide—not just a little, but as though he's giving a big yawn—quickly draw him closer and place his open mouth fully on your breast. This guiding movement should be quick but gentle. Remember that you should pull your baby to your breast, not push your breast into his mouth. If your baby's head is pushed into the breast so hard that he cannot breathe, he may become agitated or frightened and refuse to breastfeed.

If your baby is in proper nursing position, his jaws will come to-gether on your areola and his lips will seal over your breast. His chin and possibly his nose will touch your breast. (He will be able

When your baby's mouth is wide open, bring him quickly, but gently, toward your breast.

to breathe, but if you are concerned about his breathing, try lifting your breast or changing the angle of his body slightly, pulling his bottom in more closely to your body.) Helping him to latch on in a slightly asymmetric fashion, so that a bit more of the areola is in his mouth on the lower-lip side and a bit less of the areola on the upper-lip side, will position the nipple so it points toward the roof of the baby's mouth. You may feel slight discomfort when he first latches on and perhaps even for the first few sucks, but once he begins to suckle steadily you should not feel pain. *Pain beyond the first minute or so of nursing is a sign of improper latching on and should be immediately corrected through further practice and the help of a pediatrician, family physician, nurse, or lactation specialist. When pain persists throughout nursing, detach the baby by inserting your finger in the corner of his mouth to break the suction and relatch him, making sure that his mouth is wide open before latching.*

Many new mothers assume that infants are born knowing instinctively how to attach themselves to the breast and that if you

This baby is properly latched on, as his lips cover the areola and the nipple is well inside his mouth.

present your breast in the proper way he will know what to do. Certainly, some babies are capable of self-attachment, with good technique. This is most likely to occur in the first hour after birth but can be repeated later on. (Researchers have studied infants who are able to maneuver themselves from the mother's lower abdomen, where they were placed immediately after delivery, up to the nipple, where they self-attach and start suckling.) Most newborns do easily learn to latch on to the breast and soon begin the deep, regular suckling and rhythmic swallowing that typifies successful nursing. But not all babies know instinctively how to latch on: You may need to teach your baby until he experiences enough successful feedings to associate his feeding posture with the satiation of his hunger.

The key to successful latching on involves taking enough of the breast into the mouth so that the nipple is drawn to the back of the baby's mouth and his gums and tongue are compressing the areola. This suckling movement causes your baby's jaw to squeeze the milk sinuses that lay below your areola while his tongue makes a wavelike motion underneath the nipple, making your milk flow out through the tiny holes in your nipple. To achieve this, your baby's mouth must truly be open wide as he latches on. Many early nursing mistakes occur when the mother hasn't waited until her baby's jaws are about as wide as they can be before she pulls him to her breast. As a result, the baby sucks on the nipple only, a position that limits the amount of milk received and soon makes the nipple sore.

To help your baby take in a large mouthful, use your C-hold to gently compress your breast; this makes the areola narrower and the nipple stick out more so it is easier to grasp. As he latches on, his tongue should stick out a bit, cover his lower gum, and

Sliding your finger between the baby's mouth and your breast releases the suction and detaches the baby comfortably, helping you avoid nipple pain.

partially envelop the breast. His lips should curl outward and press against your breast.

If your infant doesn't manage to latch on properly the first time, gently detach him by sliding your finger into his mouth and pressing down on your breast to break the suction. Don't try to just pull him off your breast, since this could cause nipple pain. Keep practicing this latch-on technique until you and your newborn have mastered it, and don't hesitate to ask the hospital nurses and lactation specialist for help.

◆ BREASTFEEDING WITH INVERTED OR FLAT NIPPLES

As mentioned in Chapter 3, your baby may have a more difficult time latching on if your nipples are inverted or flat. Flat nipples may be almost indistinguishable from the areola or protrude only slightly with stimulation. Inverted nipples retract inward, rather than becoming erect, when the areola is compressed. They may simply have a slight dimple in the center or may recede completely instead of protruding. (See illustrations on pages 33 and 34.) If your nipples are only mildly flat, your baby may be able to attach himself to the breast without any special help. If not, try gently compressing the areola to make the nipple as erect as possible before offering it to your infant.

If this doesn't help and you continue to encounter latching-on problems, it is important to get help from a skilled pediatrician, nurse, lactation specialist, or La Leche League volunteer as soon as possible. Your infant's inability to latch on will lead to a decrease in milk supply if allowed to continue for more than a few days. Continuing to try latching on without correcting the inversion can cause painful cracks in the nipples that will make breastfeeding more uncomfortable. A lactation specialist will monitor your baby's progress, help you gain access to any necessary equipment, show you how to supplement your baby's feedings with your own expressed breastmilk when necessary, and assist you in correcting the problem as quickly and painlessly as possible. To draw your nipples out before breastfeeding, she may suggest the use of a hospital-grade electric breast pump or a manual pump, or possibly breast shells—plastic cups that press against the breast and expose the nipples.

With a specialist's assistance, your baby should soon manage to attach to the breast properly and begin to breastfeed well. This process may take from one day to several weeks—not so long compared to the year or more you hope to nurse. Some persistent cases of inverted or flat nipples may need to be addressed by a knowledgeable physician. Occasionally, some women have a severely inverted nipple on one side only and can nurse the baby on the other side. The mother will produce enough milk for her baby from only one breast, although over time, as she stops producing milk in the other breast, there will be a noticeable difference in the size of her breasts.

◆ **REFUSAL TO BREASTFEED**

If your baby continues to have a problem latching on and you don't have inverted nipples, or if he outright refuses to breastfeed almost from birth, please get help from your pediatrician or lactation specialist immediately. Your baby may be "tongue-tied"—a condition in which the membrane connecting the tongue to the floor of the mouth is too tight. Some tongue-tied babies cannot extend their tongues over the lower gumline sufficiently to latch on to the breast deeply enough. The tight membrane may need to be released (by snipping it with scissors) by a health-care provider trained in this procedure. A baby may also be unable to latch on and suckle effectively during the early feedings due to the stress of labor and delivery or medications that were given during the birth process. It's also possible that your infant's natural temperament may cause him to resist being closely held and remaining calm enough to nurse. Be careful not to hold the top of your baby's head while breastfeeding, because some babies pull away from the breast when pressure is applied to the back of their heads. In most cases—with the help of your lactation specialist, some patience, and a willingness to experiment—you will find a technique that satisfies both you and your newborn.

◆ HICCUPS, SPIT-UPS, AND BURPS

You can tell that your baby has finished nursing from one breast when he has stopped suckling, fallen asleep, or drifted off the breast. If he's not asleep, he should seem calm and relaxed. Once he's finished, you can try to burp him to expel any air he has swallowed. Breastfed babies usually swallow less air than bottle-fed infants, so he may not need to burp. Burping may ease any feeling of fullness and may wake him up a bit so that you can offer him the other breast.

Almost all babies hiccup from time to time—a phenomenon that will usually bother you more than your infant but that may distress him if he is in the middle of a feeding. As your milk supply increases, your baby may also spit up milk from time to time. This normal behavior is no cause for concern, but spit-ups and hiccups can be minimized by keeping your nursing sessions quiet and calm and changing your baby's position to help him relax.

If you choose to burp your baby after he finishes nursing on one side, hold him vertically against your body with his head over your shoulder. Place a clean cloth under his head to catch any spit-up and then *gently* pat or rub his back. If you prefer, you can perform this movement while sitting him on your lap and supporting his head with one hand or laying him across your knees on his stomach. If he hasn't burped after a few minutes, you can put him down to sleep on his back or offer him the other breast.

◆ LEARNING BY DOING

Like learning to ride a bicycle, type on a keyboard, or drive a car, it's easier to learn proper breastfeeding technique by doing it than by reading about it. Don't be put off if your first at-

A Breastfeeding Checklist: How to Tell If You're Nursing Correctly

SIGNS OF CORRECT NURSING

1. Your baby's mouth is open wide with lips curled out.

2. His chin and nose are resting against the breast.

3. He has taken as much of the areola as possible into his mouth.

4. He is suckling rhythmically and deeply, in short bursts separated by pauses.

5. You can hear him swallowing regularly.

6. Your nipple is comfortable after the first few suckles.

SIGNS OF INCORRECT NURSING

1. Your baby's head is not in line with his body.

2. He is sucking on the nipple only, instead of suckling on the areola with the nipple far back in his mouth.

3. He is sucking in a light, quick, fluttery manner rather than taking deep, regular suckles.

4. His cheeks are puckered inward or you hear clicking noises.

5. You don't hear him swallow regularly after your milk production has increased.

tempts are somewhat awkward. Remember—you and your baby are still tired from childbirth, and you, at least, are likely to feel emotionally overwhelmed. You may feel slightly uncomfortable at first with the physical sensation of breastfeeding, though that will pass. Some women feel some abdominal cramping during the first week or so of breastfeeding. This sensation, called *afterpains*, results from the release of the hormone oxytocin, which causes your uterus to shrink back to normal size and also helps your milk flow.

The fact that your breasts are producing only small quantities of colostrum at this point is also perfectly normal. Keep in mind that your milk volume will increase two to five days after birth and that babies are designed to handle this. As we pointed out in Chapter 2, newborns usually lose some weight in the days immediately after birth, only to gain it back again shortly after the mother's milk supply increases. In the meantime, please remember that what may seem complex today will seem increasingly natural and simple to you as time progresses. By keeping your long-term breastfeeding goals in mind, you can more easily meet any potential challenges presented by these first feedings and start creating a healthy life for your baby.

SUPPLY AND DEMAND: ESTABLISHING A BREASTFEEDING RHYTHM

"It was all so confusing," confessed Sheila, a new mother. "First the colostrum did not look at all like what I expected. Then Cody, my baby, kept falling asleep at the breast before he really got anything to eat. By the third day, when my milk started coming in, my breasts started to hurt from being so engorged. Cody and I couldn't seem to get into a rhythm at first where I supplied what he needed to eat and he ate what I supplied. I was pretty discouraged during our time in the hospital. I'm glad we stuck with it, though, because once we hit our stride we both really enjoyed breastfeeding."

The efficient supply-and-demand rhythm of normal breast-feeding—in which your baby's increased demand for milk spurs greater milk production from you and her diminished suckling decreases your milk supply—nearly always takes a while to establish fully and requires readjustment as your baby grows.

As your baby's suckling time increases, milk production will also increase. Her suckling stimulates nerve endings in your breast, sending a message to your brain that results in the release of the hormone prolactin. This plays a major role in stimulating milk to be created in your breasts using substances obtained from your bloodstream. As long as she continues breastfeeding, your prolactin levels surge, ensuring continued production of breast-milk. If breastfeeding is decreased—if your infant is fed on a restricted schedule or given supplemental formula, water, sugar water, or even a pacifier to satisfy her suckling urge—your milk production will decrease accordingly.

Milk production depends not only on how much your baby suckles but on how much milk she actually removes from your breast. If you were to breastfeed from only one breast, for example, the other breast would stop producing milk even though the hormones stimulated by nursing affect both breasts. (This is one reason it's a good idea to alternate which breast you use to begin nursing.) A baby who takes only the nipple into her mouth, or who otherwise attaches incorrectly and doesn't remove much milk, doesn't stimulate that breast to continue producing an adequate supply of milk. In fact, the protein contained in the residual milk remaining in the breast actually suppresses further milk production. To prevent this from happening, it's important to feed frequently from the very beginning.

The small early feedings are important to stimulate the greater milk production your baby will require in a few days' time. Newborns are born with extra water in their bodies, and weight loss occurs in the early days as the baby gets rid of this extra water, so they do not need much additional fluid. As your baby's need for fluid increases a few days after delivery, your milk will increase in water (or fluid) content, and the composition of your breastmilk will change. Over the next week or so, the protein content will decline and the fat and lactose contents increase as your milk gradually changes color from yellow to creamy white. By ten days to two weeks after childbirth, your body will have begun producing fully mature milk, in even greater abundance than before. This watery white or bluish substance contains all the nutrients your baby needs and will increase and decrease in volume according to her fluctuating demands.

Just as when learning to drive a car we sometimes push the accelerator a little too hard and then not hard enough, you may experience a hitch or two as your body adjusts to your child's appetite changes. Many mothers share Sheila's surprise at how little colostrum is available initially and how much milk fills their breasts just a few days later. This increase in milk production can lead to a tight, overfull feeling called *engorgement*. The solution to this problem is to feed your infant frequently—eight to twelve times every twenty-four hours, around the clock—even if you have to wake her to nurse. If she sleeps for stretches of longer than four hours in the first two weeks, wake her for a feeding. If she continues to sleep this long at a stretch, repeatedly falls asleep soon after starting to breastfeed, or seems listless or has a weak cry, inform her pediatrician right away. Don't wait until your baby cries to feed her; keep an eye out for early hunger cues such as smacking of

A baby's smacking lips and increased alertness and activity are early signs of hunger.

lips and increased activity. You may also need to express some milk by hand or with a pump to ease your discomfort and to soften the nipple and areola enough so that the baby can latch on.

Eventually (usually quite soon), your breastmilk production will settle down to the level your infant currently requires. During periods when she feeds more frequently—usually in response to growth spurts—your milk production will increase. (Growth spurts most commonly occur at approximately three weeks, six weeks, three months, and six months of age.) Your milk supply will decrease again when her feeding sessions decrease. You will become expert at having her suckle a little longer or more frequently when you are concerned that you may not be producing enough milk and adding a few brief "topping-off" feedings on those days when you feel somewhat engorged. This ability to tailor your milk production to both her and your needs is one of the marvels of breastfeeding.

Q & A

Is Everything Okay?

Q: *I know several women who wanted to breastfeed but had to switch to formula because they didn't have enough milk. Might this happen to me?*

A: It is rarely necessary to switch to formula because a woman is *unable* to produce enough milk for her baby. Nearly all women can breastfeed successfully, assuming they receive enough support and information. The women you know who didn't have enough milk probably did not breastfeed frequently or long enough or did not manage to get their babies latched on to the breast properly. If their babies were given supplemental feedings or a pacifier, their infants' subsequent nursing efforts may not have been strong enough to stimulate enough milk production.

The volume of breastmilk naturally fluctuates quite a bit during the first two or three weeks. The best initial solution when a newborn cries for a feeding or wakes frequently in the night to breastfeed is to continue nursing as often as possible to stimulate milk production. By using good breastfeeding techniques and focusing on exclusive breastfeeding, you will find that your baby's demand will increase your breastmilk supply. The early days and weeks are crucial in terms of getting breastfeeding off to a good start.

Q: *I was so involved in getting to know my baby and learning to breastfeed in the days following childbirth, I hardly noticed that my husband was hanging around without much to do. He was as excited about our child's arrival as I was. Is there some way to involve my husband in the early breastfeeding process?*

A: Just as your husband supported you through the birthing process, he can act as an effective coach through the early stages of breastfeeding (see Chapter 11 for more on the father's role). By remaining present when you meet with physicians, nurses, and lactation specialists, and by referring to this book, he can help you position your baby correctly when learning to nurse. He can keep an eye on the latching-on process, making sure your infant is in the proper position for getting milk. He can arrange pillows to better support your back during feeding sessions and hold and cuddle the baby when you need a rest. He may tickle your baby's foot or rub her back during a feeding to keep her stimulated if she starts to fall asleep. Or he can help burp the baby. If you gave birth by cesarean delivery, you will be especially grateful for your husband's help as you gradually recuperate from surgery. Certainly, he can play an important role by changing your baby's diapers, dressing her, playing with her, and giving her baths. By encouraging your husband to help nurture his infant in these valuable ways, you will include him in the process of helping your newborn attach in a unique way to each of her parents.

Q: *I find that breastfeeding hurts a lot for the minute or so after my baby latches on. I know how important breastmilk is for her, but the initial pain makes me want to give up. Will this situation change?*

A: Some new mothers feel more discomfort than others during different aspects of the breastfeeding process, and some women have more-sensitive nipples than others. Some feel, as you do, that the first few suckles of a breastfeeding session are uncomfortable. It may help to know that most of these sensations fade after the first couple of weeks of breastfeeding. Other mothers dislike the feeling they experience as their milk lets down, but most mothers readily adjust to this brief "pins and needles" sensation. It would be a shame to give up breastfeeding because of temporary feelings of discomfort. Hang in there for at least a week or two and then reassess how you feel. If you have *severe* pain or discomfort that does not diminish as the baby settles into nursing, ask for help with latching on and request pain medication, if needed, that's safe to take when breastfeeding.

ALREADY? HOW OFTEN TO BREASTFEED

"How often should I feed my baby?" is one of the most frequent questions new mothers ask. For the reasons outlined in the previous section, the simple answer to that question is, "As often as he's willing." Don't wait until your baby cries to put him to the breast. Crying is a late sign of hunger. He will indicate his desire to breastfeed long before he cries by smacking his lips, making suckling motions, rooting (moving his head around in search of your breast), kicking and squirming, or looking more alert. Your baby may give you such signals as often as every hour or so in the early days after birth. He should not go longer than about two to three hours during the day or four hours at night without a feeding. Even if you have to wake him up, be sure he receives eight to twelve feedings in every twenty-four-hour period. If he does not feed at first upon being awakened, wait half an hour, wake him up, and try again. Some babies will nurse even when they are not wide awake, so you don't have to awaken them completely.

Soon you will become familiar with your baby's feeding style—active and eager, sleepy and dreamy, or focused and intent. In the meantime, encourage him to feed as long as possible at each feeding. Keep him at your breast as long as he is actively suckling. Detaching a suckling baby from your breast before he's finished, or allowing him to fall asleep shortly after beginning to feed, may throw off the breastfeeding rhythm of supply and demand. Allow him to breastfeed until he seems full (at this point he will probably detach from the breast all by himself). Keep in mind that the longer your baby nurses, the higher the fat content of the milk he is drinking. Shorter, timed nursing periods may not allow him the opportunity to enjoy the full benefits of your breastmilk and may leave your breasts full of unreleased milk, making you feel engorged and uncomfortable.

Is My Newborn Getting Enough Milk?

Nearly all new mothers worry about whether their babies are properly nourished. Breastfeeding mothers cannot measure exactly how much breastmilk their newborns ingest, but they can tell in other ways whether they are getting enough to eat. Your well-nourished newborn should:

- Lose no more than seven percent of his birthweight in the first few days after birth before starting to gain weight again.

- Have one or two bowel movements per day on days one and two, with blackish, tarry stools, and at least two stools that are beginning to appear greenish to yellow on days three and four. By five to seven days, his stools should be yellow and loose, with small curds, and should number at least three to four per day. When your milk production increases, your baby will often stool with each feeding for the first month of life.

- Have six or more wet diapers per day, with nearly colorless or pale yellow urine, by five to seven days.

- Seem satisfied and happy for an average of one to three hours between feedings.

- Nurse at least eight to twelve times every twenty-four hours.

COPING WITH JAUNDICE

Many infants develop jaundice within several days after birth. A baby becomes jaundiced when bilirubin, which is produced naturally by the body, builds up faster than a newborn's liver can break it down and get rid of it in the baby's stool. Too much bilirubin makes a baby's skin and eyes look yellow. Since drinking breast-milk helps remove bilirubin through the baby's stool, babies who are not breastfeeding adequately are at greater risk of developing

Knowledge Is Power

EDUCATING YOURSELF

Unless you delivered via cesarean section or are facing some other complications relating to childbirth, your time in the hospital is likely to be quite short and full of so many consultations, visits from loved ones, and new experiences that you may feel seriously overstimulated by the time you pack to go home. Nevertheless, your hospital stay represents one of your best chances to learn more about breastfeeding while you have help available twenty-four hours a day. Take an active role in your breastfeeding education. Make sure you request the assistance of your physician, nurse, or lactation specialist the first time the baby breastfeeds. After that, continue to practice until you feel comfortable nursing. Before leaving the hospital, ask the nurse to observe your breast-feeding technique and answer the questions you have. Most hospitals now offer breastfeeding classes for new mothers, which are well worth attending; some provide videos on breastfeeding and other aspects of newborn care for use in the hospital or offer in-house television programs. In addition, the La Leche League is a phone call away. Talking to other breastfeeding mothers may provide just the information or morale boost you need. If you do not feel you're receiving the support you need from hospital staff during the days following childbirth, notify your pediatrician.

jaundice. Jaundice usually either resolves on its own or may require treatment with special lights that help break down the bilirubin. Feeding more frequently or for longer periods of time to help pass the bilirubin in the stools is almost always helpful. Certainly, there is no reason to stop breastfeeding if your baby develops jaundice of this type. In selected cases, your pediatrician might recommend a formula supplement temporarily.

Occasionally, jaundice lasts longer than two weeks. You can still usually continue breastfeeding, but sometimes your pediatrician may ask you to stop breastfeeding for a day or two. If you must interrupt breastfeeding for any reason, be sure to express your breastmilk using a quality electric breast pump (see Chapter 5) so you can keep producing milk and can restart nursing easily. Your nurse, lactation specialist, or La Leche League group can give you guidance in using a breast pump.

A NEW LIFE

On Teresa's last day in the hospital after giving birth, her pediatrician stopped by to check on the baby and observe their breastfeeding technique. After writing down Gabriel's weight and showing Teresa a more comfortable way to support her baby while nursing, he arranged for a follow-up appointment in two days and left the room. "Wow!" said Teresa's friend Linda, who had arrived to help Teresa pack. "You had a baby on Monday, and they discharge you on Wednesday. Do you really feel ready to go home?"

"I think I'm ready," Teresa said, smiling at Gabriel as she cuddled him close to her. "The nurses and the lactation specialist taught me a lot. I feel like Gabe and I really got the hang of breastfeeding this morning."

"How about help at home? Will there be someone around to take care of you?"

"Well, Gabe will be right in his cradle next to my bed, so taking care of him shouldn't be too hard," Teresa told her. "But I've got my mom coming tonight. My friend from the La Leche League will be over tomorrow to help me with breastfeeding and bring me some lunch. We're going to see the pediatrician on Friday. I have an appointment with the breastfeeding specialist at the WIC clinic next week. You know, that's where I went to the breastfeeding class before Gabriel was born."

Linda nodded. "That class seems like so long ago now, doesn't it?" she said. "Well, it looks like you're doing fine." She leaned toward the breastfeeding baby and stroked his tiny hand. "It's been quite an experience, Teresa. That Gabriel's a lucky guy."

CHAPTER 5

Special Situations

"It would have been so easy for me to quit in those early weeks when my baby was having problems, but I didn't, and I'm so glad. It was the knowledge of the benefits of breastfeeding that kept me going when I wanted to throw in the towel. My son is a year old now and has grown so big and healthy. I feel like such a success."

—Cynthia, 30, mother of Jim

"Do we have everything?" Kiyo asked her husband, Michael, as she turned toward the door of the neonatal intensive-care unit (NICU), cradling her tiny baby, Luke, in her arms. "I think so," Michael answered nervously, glancing back toward the small plastic infant bed that Luke had just vacated. The nurses in the unit smiled reassuringly at him. Luke, born eight weeks premature, had spent his first several weeks of life in the NICU. Though Luke was doing well now and was starting to gain weight nicely, his parents and his pediatrician would have to keep a close eye on him for some time to come. Both parents felt a little apprehensive now that it was finally time to take him home.

Still, it was a relief to Kiyo to know that she had given her baby the best possible start in life. Confined to bed during the latter part of her pregnancy and warned of the likelihood of a premature birth, Kiyo had researched the implications of breastfeeding a child born prematurely. She learned that the milk of the mother of a premature infant is especially beneficial for her baby, since it is custom-designed for that baby's particular stage of development. Premature infants benefit enormously from the skin-to-skin contact of breastfeeding and the immune factors and nutrients in their mothers' milk. Kiyo resolved to breastfeed Luke no matter how early he was born. When he was unable to nurse for the first week after birth, she was disappointed, but during that time she learned to use an electric breast pump, expressing breastmilk that was then fed to him through a tube. Once he was able to latch on to the breast, Kiyo breastfed him in the NICU whenever possible and continued to express milk for feedings that took place in her absence. Now, as she and her husband prepared to take their baby home, Kiyo was glad she had made the effort. At just under five pounds, Luke was a bright-eyed, lively infant, and Kiyo had managed to build up her milk production sufficiently to allow them both to enjoy the benefits of breastfeeding as he continued to grow.

Every parent naturally hopes for a normal vaginal birth without any complications, but sometimes things don't work out that way. Special birth situations may introduce challenges into the typical breastfeeding process. The best ways to deal with such challenges—and other situations that arise weeks or even months later—are to be knowledgeable about the solutions available, stay in close contact with your pediatrician, maintain a reliable and educated support network to help you in times of need, and simply make the decision to breastfeed through rough times as well as easy ones.

SPECIAL BIRTHS

Your birthing experience may affect the way you initiate breastfeeding in a number of ways. Contrary to your expectations, you may have been given anesthesia during childbirth, or your baby may have been born with a condition that makes nursing difficult. As challenging as you may find it to initiate breastfeeding under these conditions, remember that you have the advantage of well-informed breastfeeding specialists ready to assist you. It may help to know that no matter what the situation, mothers in similar circumstances have been able to breastfeed successfully.

◆ CESAREAN DELIVERY

A common circumstance encountered by women is a cesarean delivery, often referred to as a C-section, instead of a vaginal birth. The good news is that the method of delivery has little effect on your ability to nurse your baby. Your breastmilk will come in almost as readily as it would have if you had delivered vaginally. It is especially important to begin breastfeeding as soon as you are able and to continue breastfeeding your baby on a frequent basis to ensure a good milk supply. Even if you need to recover from your surgery for a few hours or as long as a day, you will be able to breastfeed as soon as you feel up to it.

Most drugs administered to mothers who give birth by cesarean delivery do not seriously affect the infant. You probably received a regional anesthetic, such as an epidural block, rather than the general anesthesia that once rendered women in childbirth unconscious. Since less regional anesthesia gets into your bloodstream than with general anesthesia, it causes less sedation for the newborn. Some newborns tend to be a bit sleepy following an epidural and may suckle with less enthusiasm at first, but no long-term negative effects on full-term babies' development or ability to breastfeed have been demonstrated. Even if you are given general anesthesia, you should be able to breastfeed as soon as you're awake enough. When you are counseled about a cesarean delivery, it is a good idea to remind the obstetrician and anesthesiologist that you intend to breastfeed.

Following cesarean delivery, your doctor will give you pain medications, initially through your IV and later in pill form, to help make you comfortable. In most cases, little of this medication passes through your breastmilk to your baby. Some pain medications may temporarily make your newborn a little sleepy, but the benefits of breastfeeding far outweigh this response. Pain interferes with the release of oxytocin, which helps your milk to flow readily for your baby, so adequate control of your pain is important. If you have any concerns about the pain medication you are being offered, speak with your doctor or lactation specialist.

Your abdominal incision may make finding a comfortable breastfeeding position a little more difficult at first. You might adjust some of the basic positions by sitting up in bed, using one or two extra pillows to support your baby on your lap and protect your incision, by lying down on your side with your baby facing you, or by using a side-sitting or football hold with enough pillows to raise your baby's head to the level of the breast (see Chapter 4). Make sure to get into a comfortable position before beginning to breastfeed, and don't be shy about asking for help. As your incision heals and you are able to move about more readily, nursing will become much easier—but expect to need some extra rest and assistance until you are fully back on your feet again.

◆ PREMATURE BIRTHS AND NEWBORN ILLNESS

Providing breastmilk for a premature or seriously ill newborn may be a challenge, but it is usually possible and it is certainly an effective way to enhance your baby's health, growth, and development. Even if your baby is unable to breastfeed at first, you can begin expressing your milk immediately after childbirth. When she is stable, she can have the milk fed to her by tube, by letting her sip the milk from a tiny cup, or perhaps from a bottle. No matter how your breastmilk is delivered to her, it provides the best nourishment possible at a time when such an advantage makes a big difference.

Mothers of premature babies produce breastmilk that is slightly different in composition, at least for the first several weeks, but this difference is designed to meet your baby's particular needs. The premature milk is higher in protein and salts and contains different types of fat to enhance the development of the baby's brain and neurologic tissues. Human milk is easier for her to digest than formula and avoids exposing her immature intes-

If your baby is born prematurely or with an illness, your expressed breastmilk may be fed to her from a tiny cup, tube, or bottle.

tinal lining to the cow's milk proteins found in premature infant formula. Premature babies who are breastfed are less likely to develop an intestinal infection than are babies who are formula-fed. Especially important is the fact that the milk you produce in the first few days contains high concentrations of antibodies to help your baby fight infection. Even if your baby cannot breastfeed yet, expressing breastmilk from the beginning will ensure that your milk supply is maintained until your baby is able to nurse.

Your first step in providing your baby with breastmilk is to enlist the support of the medical personnel who will care for your infant at the hospital. Notify your baby's pediatrician or neonatologist of your desire to breastfeed and to provide your expressed breastmilk for your baby. He can arrange to have your expressed milk fed to your baby or for you to breastfeed your infant in the neonatal nursery (many hospitals now provide private areas for nursing). Next, ask your baby's nurse or a lactation specialist in the neonatal intensive-care unit for assistance. These experienced members of your support team can show you how to assemble and use an electric breast pump, express milk efficiently, and give you advice on storing breastmilk (see Chapter 9). If you are able to directly breastfeed, they can help you adjust your nursing position to your infant's small size.

If your newborn is too small or ill to breastfeed at first, or if a birth condition prevents her from breastfeeding directly, you will find that a hospital-grade electric breast pump is the most efficient way to express milk and establish and maintain an adequate milk supply. Your hospital will provide you with a pump while you are there, and you can rent or purchase one to use at home later. The pump you use should create a milking action and not simply be a sucking device. Beginning as soon as possible after

Ask your child's pediatrician or other members of your support team for any assistance you need while breastfeeding.

your baby's birth, express your milk at regular intervals—at approximately the times when your baby would usually feed. Aim for at least six to eight times a day; this provides nipple stimulation and encourages milk production. Using a double-pump setup lets you express milk from both breasts at the same time. Most women find that the double pump produces the most milk in the least amount of time. When using the pump, continue to pump for several minutes after your milk has stopped flowing to stimulate increased milk production.

Breast massage before and during the use of the pump may help to improve your milk flow. To do this, make small, circular motions with your fingertips, starting at the outer edges of your breast near the chest wall, and slowly make your way toward the center. The massage should always be gentle to avoid producing friction on the skin surface or massaging so deeply that it causes pain.

Keep in mind that you will express only small amounts of colostrum at first, but this immune-boosting substance is extremely beneficial for your baby. Once your milk supply increases, the amount of milk you can express will probably fluctuate from day to day. As a result, you will need to increase the number of times per day you express milk to maintain an optimal milk supply. These fluctuations are normal—just more easily observed when expressing milk than when breastfeeding. Rest assured that once your baby begins breastfeeding, your milk production is likely to increase. To maximize your milk production, try to get as much rest as possible, drink adequate fluids, and minimize stress.

Your breastmilk can be fed to your baby through a tube that passes through her nose or mouth into her stomach or from a tiny cup or bottle, depending on the policies in the NICU at your hospital. Occasionally, young infants fed by bottle may start to prefer the bottle, which delivers milk faster and with less effort than feeding at the breast. Some of these babies later refuse to breastfeed—a situation called *nipple confusion* or *nipple preference.* During this period when your baby is using an alternate feeding method, you can introduce her to breastfeeding by holding her skin-to-skin against your chest whenever possible and allowing her to nuzzle and suckle at your breast. This, of course, should be done only when the neonatologist or pediatrician has given approval. Soon you may be able to progress to a nursing supplementer or other device that will deliver your expressed breastmilk from a bottle or syringe through a tiny tube that is taped next to your nipple. Eventually, your baby should begin to feed partly from the tube and partly from your breast and finally begin latching on to your breast and actively nursing.

Early breastfeeding sessions will probably be more successful if you time them for when your baby is awake and alert but calm. Experiment with different nursing positions (see Chapter 4) to discover which works best for the two of you. A premature baby often tires rather easily, so these early feedings are likely to be brief. (You can use your remaining time together to hold, rock,

A nursing supplementer delivers milk through a tube taped next to the nipple.

sing to, and play with your newborn.) Try to breastfeed as often as possible and continue to express milk for feedings in your absence. Frequent nursing and milk expression will help maintain your milk supply. An increasing number of hospitals allow mothers to room-in, or stay overnight with their babies, on the night or two prior to discharge from the NICU, enabling the mothers to start to learn their infants' round-the-clock breastfeeding rhythms and other aspects of infant care before going home. Such experience can ease the transition from hospital to home life for you and your baby.

You will naturally want to focus on making the transition from feeding your expressed breastmilk to direct breastfeeding, but understand that your hospital's medical staff wants to make sure your infant receives adequate calories and nutrition before she goes home. To achieve adequate growth and strong bones with enough calcium being deposited in them, neonatologists may enrich the diet of tiny preterm babies by adding special supplemental nutrients to the mothers' breastmilk, often in the form of commercially available human-milk fortifiers. Occasionally, the doctors may decide to feed an infant with special formulas for premature babies, sometimes alternating the formula with your breastmilk. Even if your baby is not getting feedings at all due to medical complications, continue to express your breastmilk and freeze it for later use, thus maintaining your milk production. In your conversations with the baby's doctor, be sure to reinforce your desire to breastfeed when it's medically appropriate.

After your baby is home from the hospital, you may need to keep using your breast pump for at least a month (especially after short feedings). This lets you store breastmilk for extra feedings and maintain an adequate milk supply, especially as your baby grows and his needs increase. Attempt to nurse whenever your baby shows an interest—even if it's every hour or hour and a half during the early weeks. Finally, have your breastfeeding technique rechecked by your pediatrician or a lactation specialist shortly after your baby's homecoming.

Caring for and learning to breastfeed a premature or ill newborn is emotionally taxing for any new mother. It's a good idea to contact any support groups in your area that specialize in your baby's condition. Other mothers are often the most valuable sources of information. Make sure, too, that your partner and other family members understand the enormous advantages of breastfeeding a preterm baby or an ill hospitalized newborn. The emotional and practical support of your loved ones will go a long way in helping you achieve your breastfeeding goals.

◆ TWINS AND OTHER MULTIPLES

Giving birth to multiples is certainly not a "problem" in the traditional sense, but if you are the new mother of twins, triplets, or more multiples, you may worry about how you will manage to breastfeed them all. If you have twins, you can breastfeed them at

You can breastfeed twins simultaneously. This mother is using both the cradle hold and the football hold.

the same time by holding one baby at each side in a football hold (see Chapter 4) or by cradling both infants in front of you with their bodies crossing each other.

You may need to express breastmilk as well as breastfeed, since multiples are frequently born prematurely and require special care. A hospital-grade electric breast pump will help maximize your milk supply until your babies have fully adjusted to breastfeeding and are gaining weight appropriately. Your lactation specialist, local Mothers of Twins club, or La Leche League can offer advice on where to find a pump and provide other helpful information. Meanwhile, be sure that your pediatrician monitors your babies' weight to make sure each is getting an adequate amount of breastmilk to ensure proper weight gain.

If you have triplets, you can breastfeed them as well. But do not be discouraged if your pediatrician recommends supplementing feedings with formula. You might find nursing two of your babies at a time and giving formula or expressed breastmilk to the third works the best. At the next feeding, give the formula to a different baby. All three (or more) babies should have a chance to breastfeed. And it's especially important for you to get adequate rest and have good help with household chores and baby care to establish and maintain a milk supply for all of your babies.

CONSIDERING YOUR OWN HEALTH

For some new mothers, concerns about breastfeeding revolve less around their babies' physical condition than their own. Since some infectious diseases can be transmitted to the baby through human milk, you will certainly want to discuss your medical history with your doctor and your baby's pediatrician. The American Academy of Pediatrics (AAP) and the Centers for Disease Control and Prevention (CDC) advise mothers in the United States who are infected with HIV (human immunodeficiency virus) not to breastfeed, since the virus may be passed in the breastmilk to their infant. They may, however, feed their babies donor breastmilk, which has been obtained from mothers who are free from HIV or other infectious diseases and processed by a donor milk bank.

If you are infected with hepatitis B, your baby should receive the vaccination for hepatitis B—along with hepatitis immune globulin (HBIG)—as soon as possible after birth. Giving these two injections within twelve hours after delivery is highly effective in preventing the spread of hepatitis B from mother to infant and is recommended whether you are breastfeeding or not. Hepatitis B virus has been detected in human milk, but breastfeeding has not been shown to increase the risk of infection to the baby. The AAP states that maternal infection with hepatitis B is compatible with breastfeeding and there is no need to delay initiation of breastfeeding until the infant is immunized for hepatitis B.

Both the AAP and the Centers for Disease Control state that infection with hepatitis C is compatible with breastfeeding. Though an infant can be infected with hepatitis C during pregnancy or delivery, breastfeeding does not increase his risk of infection.

Other types of infections need to be evaluated by your obstetrician, pediatrician, or family physician, but few will prevent breastfeeding. This is true even when the infection or inflammation involves the breast itself—as in the case of mastitis, an infection of a segment of the breast. This condition is typically treated with antibiotics, frequent breastfeeding or expression of milk with a pump, adequate fluids, pain medication, and rest.

If you have tuberculosis (TB), you may breastfeed if you are currently taking medication. Mothers with untreated TB at the time of delivery should not breastfeed until they have started appropriate drug treatment and they are no longer infectious. If you've had a positive TB skin test but a normal chest X ray, talk to your doctor to see if you need to be treated with any medication, but you can breastfeed.

◆ CANCER

If you have been diagnosed with breast cancer in the past and have been treated for it, you may be concerned about the effects of breastfeeding on you and your baby. Previous breast cancer does not mean that you cannot breastfeed your baby. If you have had a mastectomy, you can feed from the remaining breast. If you have had a tumor removed from your breast or radiation treatments, you can still try feeding from that breast. You may find that your milk production is less, however. Always discuss your breastfeeding options with your physician.

What Is That?

DISCOVERING A LUMP
WHILE BREASTFEEDING

Some women get plugged milk ducts, which are painful or sensitive to touch but can be easily treated (see Chapter 8). And lactating breasts may feel lumpy. However, do not ignore a lump or bump in your breast that develops during lactation and does not go away with gentle massage and breastfeeding or milk expression. A lump may represent the first signs of breast cancer and must be evaluated by your physician. Mammograms are more difficult for a radiologist to interpret during lactation. Nevertheless, breast self-exams and annual physician breast exams should continue throughout the lactation period.

It is possible to continue breastfeeding while undergoing mammograms and other diagnostic procedures, including ultrasounds and biopsies, though a temporary interruption is sometimes necessary. If you have a lump or cyst removed, it is generally safe to breastfeed afterward. Monitor your baby's weight gain, however, as surgical incisions may sever milk ducts and nerves related to milk production and release.

◆ BREAST SURGERY

In the past, concerns have arisen about the safety of breast-feeding after breast enlargement with breast implants. But there is no evidence that silicone breast implants cause any harm to the baby, and the newer saline (salt-water-filled) implant devices do not cause any problems either. In most cases, plastic surgery to enlarge the breasts should not interfere significantly with your ability to breastfeed—provided the nipples have not been moved and no milk ducts have been cut. With any previous breast surgery, however, the baby will need to be monitored carefully to make sure that he is getting enough milk.

Plastic surgery to reduce the size of breasts (breast reduction) is more likely to interfere with breastfeeding, especially if the nipples were removed and then replaced during the course of the surgery—resulting in the cutting of ducts or nerves. Many women who have had this type of breast surgery are able to breastfeed, however. If you have had any surgical procedure on your breast, even a biopsy, make sure that your doctor knows this, but by all means begin breastfeeding, making sure that your pediatrician or family physician closely monitors your infant to make sure he is receiving adequate breastmilk.

◆ MAINTAINING YOUR MILK SUPPLY

If you are temporarily unable to breastfeed because of a severe illness or while taking contraindicated medications, keep up your milk supply by expressing milk either by hand, with a manual breast pump (see Chapter 9), or with an electric pump (see Chapter 10). Obviously, this process is not the same as actual breastfeeding, and it may seem pointless if the breastmilk needs to be discarded while your baby receives previously expressed milk, donor breastmilk, or formula. But remember that while your illness will not last long, breastfeeding may continue for months or years. By using a pump to maintain your milk production, you can ensure an ongoing breastfeeding relationship with your child after you recover and for a long time to come. In rare instances, when the mother is unable to pump because of severe illness, hospital staff can express milk to maintain comfort, decrease the risk of developing a breast infection, and ensure continued milk production.

◆ GETTING HELP AND INFORMATION

No matter what your concerns may be about breastfeeding—whether your baby was born prematurely, you are worried about the effects of past breast surgery, or you wonder whether a disease or infection may be passed to your child through your breastmilk—it is vital to communicate your complete medical history to your child's pediatrician and your doctor, and be sure to emphasize your desire to breastfeed if at all possible. Since some medical professionals may not be as knowledgeable about the potential benefits of breastfeeding ill or very premature infants, you may need to provide them with information supporting your position. (Relevant information is available on the AAP Website www.aap.org or from the La Leche League. See "Breastfeeding Resources" for contact information.) If direct breastfeeding does not appear to be a possibility now or in the future, ask your pediatrician to help you explore the best alternatives—including expressing your breastmilk for tube- or bottle-feeding; combining breastmilk with additional formula-feeding; or feeding your infant breastmilk obtained from a milk bank. The hospital where you give birth should provide you with a hospital-grade electric breast pump if you require one while you're there, but you will need a pump of your own once you're home. The hospital lactation specialist can help you locate one.

MEDICATIONS: WHAT TO TAKE, AND WHAT NOT TO TAKE, WHILE BREASTFEEDING

After delivery, many women are relieved that they no longer have to worry that taking a pain reliever or cold pill may negatively affect their fetus's development. Still, if you are breastfeeding and plan to take any kind of drug—whether prescription or over-the-counter—be sure to get the approval of your obstetric or pediatric health-care provider. Most medications are safe to take during breastfeeding, but a few can be dangerous for your baby—and they are not necessarily the same ones that were dangerous during pregnancy. Your doctor is the best source of the most up-to-date information on which medications are safe for you at this time.

Much is still unknown regarding long-term effects of various kinds of medications. For this reason, it's important to take medication only when absolutely necessary while breastfeeding, to use the safest drug, and to take the lowest dose possible. When possible, use short-acting drugs rather than sustained-release varieties. Short-acting drugs are best taken immediately after a nursing session, while longer-acting medications should be taken just after your baby's last evening feeding or before his longest sleep period. When taking any medication, watch closely for reactions in your baby, including loss of appetite, diarrhea, sleepiness, excessive crying, vomiting, or skin rashes. Call your baby's pediatrician immediately if any of these symptoms appear. In the event that your doctor needs to prescribe for you a potentially harmful drug for a short time, you can express and store breastmilk ahead of time and then express and discard the milk containing the drug until it is cleared out of your body. The length of time required to clear the drug from your system varies based on the particular medication, but your doctor or pharmacist should advise you about this.

◆ BIRTH CONTROL

Frequent, exclusive breastfeeding (no water, juice, formula, or other supplements for the baby), including at least one night feeding, significantly reduces the chance of your becoming

Home Cures

HOMEOPATHIC AND HERBAL MEDICINES

Many Americans are accustomed to turning to homeopathic remedies to treat routine illnesses, particularly when they are concerned about side effects associated with more mainstream medicines. However, just because a remedy is "natural" doesn't mean it's safe for breastfeeding women or their babies. In many cases, very little scientific research has been done regarding the implications of using such cures while nursing. In the United States, the Food and Drug Administration (FDA) does not regulate homeopathic, herbal, or natural remedies, meaning that the government does not oversee these products for purity or make sure that no toxic substances are present. Certain substances are known to create such negative effects as increased blood pressure and reduced breastmilk supply when taken in large quantities. It's best to treat homeopathic remedies just as you would any medicine: Refrain from ingesting herbs or other homeopathic medications (aside from commercially produced herbal teas) unless your family physician, obstetrician, or pediatrician has approved them. Take approved substances in the smallest doses possible and carefully observe your baby for any negative reactions. Make sure your doctor and your baby's pediatrician are aware of anything you are taking.

pregnant again during the first six months after birth. However, after about six weeks you can begin using contraceptives if your milk supply is firmly established and you have discussed the issue with your obstetrician or gynecologist. While no harmful effects on infants have been demonstrated when mothers use hormonal contraceptives, research has shown that birth-control pills with high doses of estrogen may decrease milk supply. Progestin-only pills (sometimes referred to as mini-pills) are least likely to interfere with breastfeeding, although they have increased side effects for the mother. Effects vary from woman to woman and with the type of pill, so discuss the possible ramifications with your doctor before you begin taking contraceptives. You might also consider using condoms, a diaphragm, or a cervical cap and spermicide instead, since these forms of birth control are least likely to interfere with your milk supply.

STARTING OVER: RELACTATING AND RESUMING BREASTFEEDING

Mothers stop breastfeeding for a variety of reasons. Some may have decided against breastfeeding initially or experienced breastfeeding problems that led to unplanned early weaning. A separation from a baby due to hospitalization or other causes may have led to a decreasing milk supply despite pumping. An unaddressed imbalance in the breastfeeding rhythm or stress may have affected your milk let-down. Whatever the reason for the cessation of breastfeeding, it is sometimes possible to begin again—to *relactate*—if not always to completely nourish your child, at least enough to maintain the breastfeeding relationship. This may be especially important if you stopped breastfeeding only to find that your baby did not tolerate infant formulas.

Relactation works best if you either gave birth fairly recently (particularly if your child is less than three months old) or if your milk supply has been low or nonexistent for only a short period of time. While doctors may prescribe such drugs as metoclopramide to adoptive mothers who have not previously breastfed (see box on next page) or to women attempting to relactate, the baby's frequent suckling and other forms of nipple stimulation, such as an electric breast pump, are critical to establishing or reestablishing milk supply.

If you are attempting to relactate, nurse your baby frequently, whenever he shows such hunger cues as a pursed mouth, sucking motions, or increased activity or alertness. You may need to nurse eight to ten or even more times per day, with two or more night feedings, for about fifteen to twenty minutes per session. If your baby is not eager to nurse as you are building your milk supply, provide him with positive reinforcement by using a nursing supplementer to provide formula or expressed or donor breastmilk. You should also stimulate your breasts with breast message and a good-quality breast pump.

Don't expect this process to lead to instant results. Your baby may resist nursing for a week to two before he settles back down to breastfeeding, and it may take weeks for your milk supply to increase. To improve your chances of relactating, try to keep your nursing sessions relaxed and pleasurable for both you and your child. Drink enough liquids, and try to maintain an adequate diet. Ask for help from your obstetric or pediatric provider, La Leche League volunteer, or lactation specialist, and support from family members and friends who may have experienced the same process.

Relactation does not always mean a return to exclusive breastfeeding. Since your breastmilk production may well be lower than it was originally, you may need to supplement your baby's nutritional intake with breastmilk from a donor milk bank, formula, or solid foods if he is older than six months. If he is not allergic to cow's milk, then it may be given after one year of age. Meanwhile, it is crucial to monitor his weight gain and other signs that he is getting adequate calories and nutrition. Be sure that your pediatrician or family physician is aware of your breastfeeding situation and bring your child in for checkups as requested.

Inducing Lactation in Adoptive Mothers

A growing number of adoptive mothers are interested in breast-feeding their babies through induced lactation.

No drugs specifically designed to induce or enhance lactation have yet been approved by the FDA. However, a few medications typically prescribed for other reasons, such as the drug metoclopramide, have also been shown to stimulate or enhance milk production. Such medications must be prescribed by a physician and do have side effects, so your doctor will want to review your medical history before prescribing them. Herbal medications, available either in capsules or in teas, have been used by mothers in the United States and other countries to stimulate or increase milk supply. Ask your doctor or lactation specialist about herbal medications before considering their use. (Note that herbal medications are not regulated in the United States for content, purity, or possible contaminants.)

Any medication you use must be accompanied by regular nipple stimulation with a breast pump every two to three hours. Once your baby has arrived, he can be encouraged to suckle at the breast, initiating a breastfeeding relationship while further stimulating milk production. While there is no way to predict whether your milk production will reach sufficient levels to fully satisfy your baby's needs, many adoptive mothers happily breastfeed with the aid of a nursing supplementer that provides donor breastmilk or formula.

WHAT A BIG BOY!
THE REWARDS OF PERSISTENCE

"Where is that little grandson of mine?" Kiyo's mother-in-law excitedly asked as she entered the house, hardly hesitating to give her son and daughter-in-law a quick embrace. "I haven't seen Luke in six months, and Grandma wants a kiss."

"He's in here, Donna," Kiyo said, exchanging a grin with her husband. "Playing with the blocks you sent him. See?"

Donna spied her only grandson sitting in the corner of the living room, and her face lit up with surprise. "He's so *big*!" she exclaimed. "What happened? He must have gained twenty pounds since he was born."

"No, just ten," Michael said proudly, picking up his son. Luke clung to the block he was holding, gazing alertly at this stranger who had such a huge grin. "Ah," he said authoritatively, throwing the block to the floor.

"Oh, and a genius too," his grandmother commented, reaching for him and taking him in her arms. "Just like his mommy, I guess," she added with a wink at Kiyo. "Come on, big guy. Let's go sit down in the kitchen. I've got a surprise for you."

Smiling, Kiyo followed her family into the kitchen. Luke did look extraordinarily healthy and alert now, she reflected—especially compared to how tiny he seemed after birth. It was hard to believe that a baby's development could proceed so quickly, especially after such a difficult start. Kiyo was convinced that plenty of love and attention, along with the nutritional and health benefits of breastmilk, played an important role. In retrospect, Kiyo was more glad than ever that she had been determined to breastfeed Luke, even though she'd needed to convince her family that breastfeeding was best for her premature son. The result, after all, was a healthy, happy little boy, a proud father, and a mother who knew she did her very best for her child.

CHAPTER 6

Going Home

*"Breastfeeding is an art, and like anything new it takes a
little time to make it work smoothly. New mothers and babies
must learn how to make a nursing relationship successful.
The only way to succeed is determination."*

—Linda, 28, mother of Melody

"Grandma! They're here!" Ayiesha and her husband, Paul, could
hear Jason, their four-year-old son, announcing their arrival even
before they opened their front door. Ayiesha cradled her newborn daughter, Sophie, a little more securely in her arms as she
entered her living room, preparing for the physical onslaught of
her delighted preschooler. "Let me see her!" Jason said, pulling
back the blanket to reveal Sophie's wide eyes and puckered
frown. "She looks like you, Daddy." As Sophie began to cry
loudly, he added, "She sounds like you too!"

"Can I get you anything, honey?" Ayiesha's mother asked, en-
tering the room and smiling down at the baby. She'd already seen
Sophie during several visits to the hospital and was now eager to
welcome her daughter and her new granddaughter home.

"No thanks, Mom," Ayiesha said, sinking into a favorite armchair. "Sophie's hungry, I think. I'll just feed her and then we can
talk." As Paul went off to their bedroom to get the footstool
Ayiesha used when nursing Jason as a baby, Ayiesha lifted up her
shirt, unfastened the front flap on her nursing bra, and made sure

that Sophie was correctly latched on. Ayiesha was not surprised to see that Jason was watching attentively. The two of them had talked a bit during her pregnancy about how she would feed his new sister—the same way that she had once fed him. They'd read a few children's books about a new baby in the house and talked about the many different feelings Jason might have about Sophie. Ayiesha understood that her son's interest now sprang from his natural curiosity about the breastfeeding process. She had worried that Jason would feel jealous when he first saw Sophie nursing, but for now he seemed only interested in, and even charmed by, the scene he was witnessing.

"What's she drinking?" he asked in a hushed voice as Sophie suckled at her mother's breast.

Ayiesha knew that he knew the answer but wanted to hear it confirmed anyway. "She's drinking Mommy's special milk," she told him with a smile. "It makes her grow big and strong and helps keep her from getting sick. This is how you used to eat when you were a baby."

The answer seemed to satisfy Jason, because he abruptly turned and dashed into the kitchen. "Grandma!" he shouted. "Can I have one of the cookies we made for Mommy today?"

A HEALTHY START

Whether or not you have other children waiting for you, your return home will be a momentous occasion for you, your partner, and certainly for your baby. You will begin or continue your family life together, and all the plans and expectations you have created for this time will—hopefully—start to fall into place. If this is your first child, you will need time to learn how to integrate breastfeeding into your everyday life. You will want to familiarize yourself with your baby's unique nursing style, respond to her changing feeding rhythms and needs, and learn how to meet your own needs for sleep, proper nutrition, and adult companionship in the process. If you have other children at home, you will need to do this while caring for the rest of your family. No matter what your home situation, you will want to allow time to adjust to your new circumstances, regain your strength and energy, practice the nursing techniques and positions you've recently learned, and get to know your new baby. This may sound overwhelming, but you will learn how to handle it. For most women the pleasures of breastfeeding—knowing they are giving their babies the best possible introduction to life, feeling the closeness to their newborns that nursing brings, and experiencing motherhood in this most natural of ways—make the effort more than worthwhile.

A SPECIAL PLACE FOR A SPECIAL TIME: ESTABLISHING A NURSING ROUTINE

It is such a joy to observe an infant's responses to the world into which he was so recently born. As you watch your newborn gaze in wonder at the people and objects around him, nestle against you with a whimper of pleasure, and occasionally startle with panic or fear, you may feel that you're experiencing many of the same emotions yourself. During the first days and weeks at home with a new baby, you may swing between feelings of joy and uncertainty, confidence and confusion, excitement and exasperation. These are all very natural and expected feelings. If your emotional responses during the postpartum period are more extreme than you expected or feel you can handle, you should notify your physician. In general, the simpler and more predictable you can keep your daily routine, as you continue getting to know your infant and familiarizing yourself with breastfeeding, the better for you and your family.

Though one of the great advantages of breastfeeding is its adaptability—you can feed your baby practically anywhere without equipment and without delay—you might find that choosing one or two favorite places for breastfeeding at first will make your

You Feed the Baby with Your Body?

MANAGING OLDER SIBLINGS

Many women who breastfeed their newborns wonder how their older children will respond to nursing sessions and worry about how to keep older siblings occupied during frequent early breastfeeding sessions. It's safe to assume that all your children will show a healthy curiosity about this amazing and beautiful manner of feeding a brand-new baby. As long as you explain the nursing process in simple language and maintain a matter-of-fact approach to their questions and their desire to watch the baby breastfeed, such "family time" may turn out to be a positive and educational experience for all.

Don't be surprised if your older children tend to hover nearby during nursing sessions or even try to climb into your lap. Include them if you can by talking about how you used to breastfeed them (if you did), giving them a little hug with your free arm, telling them a story, or watching while they draw you a picture, work in a workbook, or play with a toy. You might also read one of the children's books about breastfeeding listed in "Breastfeeding Resources." Some mothers find that nursing sessions are wonderful times to listen to recordings of music or children's stories with their babies' siblings. In this way, nursing time can be used to draw closer to all the children, not just the new one. Older children may also be grateful for the chance to express the feelings of closeness that breastfeeding inspires by folding laundry nearby, getting you a glass of water, holding the baby while you prepare to nurse, or otherwise contributing to their family's care.

If your toddler or preschooler asks if she can try nursing, the choice is obviously yours. In most cases, a child who is no longer breastfed may find the experience too strange to try more than once. She will probably not remember how to nurse and will run off, satisfied, after a quick experiment.

If you already have a nursing toddler who may not want to relinquish the breast when your new baby enters the family, or if you feel that this is not the time to begin weaning, you may decide to *tandem nurse*—breastfeed both the toddler and the newborn. If so, be sure to inform your newborn's pediatrician of your decision so your infant's growth can be monitored more closely. Keep in mind that while the older child can receive foods and liquids from other sources, your infant depends entirely on your breastmilk for her nutrition. Therefore, you should offer the breast to your infant first, and nurse your older child only after your infant has had her fill. Also watch your own nutrition and energy levels more closely. You will need to eat well enough to support the production of extra breastmilk and get the additional rest necessary to handle the extra demands on your body. Your baby's pediatrician will be aware of all of these issues and can help you deal with them. You may wonder whether the newborn will still receive the advantages of colostrum during tandem nursing. Analysis of mother's milk shows that a mother who delivers a newborn does produce colostrum and milk designed to meet the needs of the newborn, even though the mother is still nursing a toddler. This offers the desired advantages for the newborn, but no adverse consequences for the older child.

adjustment easier. During the day, you might opt for a sofa or chair in the living room or kitchen, since this allows you to take part in family life as you nurse. Some new mothers find that breastfeeding in bed, with plenty of pillows for support and their baby's bassinet waiting close by, allows the baby to drift off comfortably to sleep at the end of the nursing session and makes it easier for the mother to nap.

Transitioning from nursing at the hospital to nursing at home is an enriching and rewarding experience.

Nursing mothers in many cultures sleep with their babies until they wean. The American Academy of Pediatrics, however, has expressed concern that bed sharing and co-sleeping may be hazardous under certain conditions. Bed sharing is a particular concern if the mother is obese or is using any substances that may alter her state of arousal, such as mind-altering drugs or excessive alcohol. If you decide to let your infant sleep in your bed, be sure *never* to place him in a facedown position. Avoid soft surfaces, loose pillows, or loose covers, and move the bed away from the wall and other furniture to keep your baby from becoming trapped. Never put your baby to sleep on a waterbed. Consider moving him to his bassinet, on his back, after breastfeeding and before you drift off to sleep.

Once you've picked a couple of locations for breastfeeding,

make sure that such essentials as baby wipes and diapers are within reach before you start nursing. Keep a bottle of water or something else to drink nearby for yourself, as nursing mothers should drink plenty of water or other noncaffeinated fluids to avoid thirst. If you have older children, a basket of toys, workbooks, or audio recordings can keep you from having to get up in the middle of a breastfeeding session. You might also keep a pad and pencil within reach to track your baby's feedings (you can also use the breastfeeding record in the appendix). Finally, while studies have shown that eye contact and other communication during feedings benefits your infant's brain development (and is rewarding for you too), you may want to keep a magazine or the television remote control within reach for those times when he falls asleep in your arms. Of course, you won't necessarily need every one of these items, nor do you need to create a formal "nursing area" to breastfeed successfully, but thinking ahead about what you might want nearby can make life more manageable in the early days.

◆ FINDING TIME ALONE

Once you have started breastfeeding at home, you may feel as though you never stop—particularly during the first week or two. Though breastfed babies exhibit a wide range of normal feeding patterns (and these patterns frequently differ even day to day), many babies begin feeding every hour or two as they learn to suckle effectively and as your milk supply becomes established. While not all of these sessions will be full feedings (you may have a baby who enjoys "snacking" frequently), healthy newborns breastfeed about eight to twelve times per day—that is, once every two or three hours on average. In many cases, daytime feedings may be less than two hours apart, leaving time for somewhat longer periods of sleep at night. It is easy to see, then, why new mothers who breastfeed postpone plans to send out baby announcements, finish the nursery, or entertain visitors until about two to three weeks after birth. By focusing on your relationship with your newborn, you can make sure that your milk supply is established, your breastfeeding relationship is securely in place, you baby is receiving the nutrition he needs, and the two of you are communicating well.

Of course, it's not often easy to enjoy a private "honeymoon" with one's newborn. The baby's father naturally wants to establish a relationship with his infant and to spend time with you. Friends and relatives are eager to see the baby and offer all kinds of parenting advice. Your other children will not only want to play with the baby but may need and demand more attention as they watch you tending to their new sibling. Of course, such needs must be met to some degree. But just as you needed to look out for your newborn's needs in the hospital, it's important to limit your interactions, as well as your baby's, with others for the two or three weeks it takes to establish your daily rhythm. Restrict visitors to

Some nursing sessions provide a great opportunity to spend time with the entire family.

Home, but Not Alone

GETTING THE HELP YOU REALLY NEED

Everyone loves a newborn, and you may find yourself besieged with well-wishers once you have returned home with your baby. Support is always welcome, of course, but when it interferes with your developing breastfeeding relationship (when a relative offers to give the baby a bottle of formula, juice, or water, for example, so that you can "get some rest"), you will need to excuse yourself and your infant from the celebration or redirect your visitors' energy. Try asking helpers who want to feed the baby to prepare meals for the family instead, spend time with older children, do the laundry, or entertain other visitors while you and your baby take a nap. If your mother or mother-in-law longs to cuddle her new grandchild, ask her to hold the baby while you take a shower or get dressed. If you find you are hav-ing trouble with breastfeeding or other new parenting skills, a visitor who is an experienced breastfeeding mother may be able to help you enormously during this period. If you know that your helper's knowledge in this area is limited, however, or she does not agree with your philosophy regarding breastfeeding, quietly turn to your "official" support system (your child's pediatrician or family physician, your La Leche League volunteer, or a lactation specialist) instead. Of course, you can still appreciate and thank your friend for her efforts.

the one or two people who you think will really be able to help with the household management (while leaving much of the baby-cuddling to you), and schedule visits with others for a month from now or even later. Use a telephone answering machine to screen calls so that you can get enough sleep and save your energy for your baby. As far as sleep goes, whenever your newborn sleeps, consider napping yourself instead of trying to get household chores done. If you have hired a professional baby nurse or doula (a helper who "mothers the mother so she can mother her baby"), make sure she focuses on freeing you up from household and social obligations, so that you have little to worry about besides caring for yourself and your infant, establishing a breastfeeding rhythm, eating well and getting enough sleep. Ask your doula or your partner to help with the other children.

SETTLING IN: THE FIRST FEW WEEKS OF BREASTFEEDING

The first weeks of breastfeeding are a fascinating time of transition for you as well as your baby. During this time you will learn what it feels like to breastfeed correctly, how to recognize your baby's hunger signals, and how to know when your let-down reflex or milk ejection has occurred (see Chapter 2). You will learn whether your baby is a frequent snacker or prefers less frequent but longer meals, whether nursing tends to put her to sleep or to stimulate her, and whether she enjoys pausing occasionally to exchange looks with you or focuses entirely upon nursing until she's had her fill. She will not always breastfeed in the same way, of course—just as you will not always be in the same mood each time you nurse. But you will begin to respond to discernible trends in breastfeeding behavior. As you do so, the two of you will gradually grow more comfortable together, respond to each other's signals more effectively, and develop a unique breastfeeding rhythm.

Ideally, by the time you arrive home your baby will already have learned to latch on to the breast properly. (If she hasn't, it's very important to address this issue immediately by reviewing the instructions in Chapter 4 and asking for help from your baby's pediatrician, your La Leche League volunteer, or a lactation specialist.) Your newborn may even prefer one breast at this point, tending to nurse longer on one than on the other. It is a good idea to let her nurse as long as she wants. Keep in mind that once your mature milk comes in, its content changes during the course of a single breastfeeding—from the somewhat watery *foremilk* to the creamier, fat-rich *hindmilk*, which, like any good dessert, leaves your baby feeling content and sleepy. By allowing your baby to nurse until she's satisfied (once she's latched on properly), you can ensure that she will receive all the benefits of breastmilk.

Even if she clearly prefers one breast over the other, however, it's important to alternate the breast you offer *first* with each breastfeeding session. This ensures that a full milk supply is stimulated for both breasts and that as much milk as possible has been removed from each. At first, to remember which breast to start with, move a safety pin from one side of your nursing bra to the other after each feeding. Later on you will know which breast feels fuller and start the next feeding there.

◆ IS SHE EATING WELL?

As you feed your baby, continue to look for the signs of correct nursing. In addition to making sure she is latched on properly, with her mouth around as much of the areola as possible, you should hear her swallow as her mouth fills with milk. During the first few days she may not swallow as often, since the volume of the colostrum she is ingesting is still low. After the second to fifth day following childbirth, however, your milk will have increased in volume and your baby should be swallowing after every one or two sucks once the milk has let down. While she is nursing, you may see some milk escaping from around her lips or notice that milk is dripping from your other breast. These are good signs that your let-down reflex is working properly (see below) and your body is producing the breastmilk your baby needs. After a nursing session, your infant should appear content and satisfied. If she continues to fuss, she may want to return to the breast for more milk, need to burp, or may simply want to be cuddled or played with.

It is important during this early period to breastfeed your baby whenever she shows signs of hunger, rather than delaying in an effort to stick to a set schedule. Don't wait for her to cry for a feeding; bring her to the breast as soon as you see increased activity or alertness. Keep in mind that the more frequently your baby nurses, the more she will stimulate your milk production and the more easily and quickly the two of you will reach a satisfactory balance of milk supply and demand. If your baby tends to sleep for long periods or is simply undemanding, you may need to encourage her to feed more often than she would naturally. Wake her up for a feeding after four hours of sleep, initiate breastfeeding every few hours whether or not she acts hungry on her own, and continue nursing for at least ten minutes (and preferably longer) to ensure that she gets plenty of milk. It is also best to avoid pacifiers for at least the first month or so to encourage your baby to do all her suckling at the breast.

◆ CHECKING HER DIAPER

Some of the best signs that your baby is breastfeeding successfully can be found in her diaper. As your milk supply becomes more abundant, your breastfeeding baby will wet more diapers per day. By five to seven days after birth, she should be wetting her diaper at least six to eight times in a twenty-four-hour period. You may have to look closely to tell whether a highly absorbent disposable diaper is wet. Comparing the weight of a fresh diaper to the one you are removing can help you decide if the baby has urinated in the diaper. Coinciding with the increase in your milk volume (generally after the second to fifth

day), you should also check that the urine is colorless or pale yellow—not dark yellow or red- or pink-speckled. (The latter are
signs of highly concentrated urine, which may be normal in the
first few days after delivery but later could indicate that your
baby is not getting enough milk.) Once your milk volume increases, your infant should also pass about three or four bowel
movements each day. These stools will consist of loose, yellow
curds—no longer the tarry-black stool of the first few days—and
much of the normal watery stool may be absorbed into a diaper,
leaving what appears to be a stain. Some infants pass a yellow
stool after each feeding at this point, and this is considered perfectly normal during the early weeks. After about a month the
number of bowel movements will start to decrease. Babies older
than one month will sometimes go for days or even a week or
more without passing a stool. This, too, is normal, as long as she
still feeds eagerly, is gaining weight well, has a soft tummy, and
has a soft, usually large stool when she does have one. Anytime
you have concerns about your baby's stool or urination patterns,
consult your pediatric health-care provider.

◆ WEIGHT GAIN

While diapers can provide important indications that a baby
is not getting enough to eat, your baby's weight gain remains the
most reliable sign of breastfeeding success. A breastfeeding baby
who is getting enough milk will gain weight, while a baby who is
nursing inadequately will not gain as well or may even lose
weight. Most babies lose up to seven percent of their birthweight
in the first few days after birth (with larger babies tending to lose
more weight than smaller ones), but this weight loss should stop
once your milk production increases, beginning around the second to fifth day following childbirth. At that time, your infant
should start regaining her lost weight right away. She will usually
exceed her birthweight by fourteen days after birth. From about
her fifth day of life through her third month, she should gain
one-half ounce to one ounce per day, or one-half to one pound

every two weeks. Your pediatrician will weigh your baby during the initial breastfeeding checkup, a couple of days after you return home from the hospital.

◆ YOUR BREASTS

Your breasts can also provide a great deal of information about how well your breastfeeding relationship with your baby is progressing. As we pointed out in Chapter 2, your breasts should increase in size and feel heavier about two to five days after delivery—a feeling that tells you your transitional milk has come in. At feeding times, your breasts may become so full and firm that your baby has trouble latching on correctly. In this case, you may need to hand-express or pump a little milk for a few minutes to soften them (see Chapter 9). If you have any trouble managing this or your baby still cannot latch on, ask your pediatrician, lactation specialist, or an experienced friend for help right away. It is important for your baby to continue to breastfeed as frequently as she wants to during this period when your level of milk production is being established.

Once your baby latches on properly and begins to nurse, you may feel the tingly pins-and-needles sensation of the milk let-down or milk-ejection reflex. This reflex—a physiological response to your baby's stimulation of your nipples while feeding—causes your milk to flow more plentifully, providing your baby with the abundant milk she needs. The milk-ejection reflex should be noticeable to most mothers by about two weeks after delivery. In the early days after childbirth, when oxytocin is released in your body in response to your baby's feeding, you may also notice cramping in your lower abdomen. In fact, some women primarily note the uterine contractions, as opposed to the squeezing sensation in their breasts, in the early postpartum days. The cramping is a good sign, even though it may produce temporary discomfort. These contractions of the muscles of your uterus help it return to its pre-pregnancy size, preventing excessive uterine bleeding.

Once your baby has nursed fully on each breast, your breasts will feel soft again—letting you know that your baby has had an adequate feeding. By about two to three weeks after birth, your breasts will feel not quite as excessively firm between feedings, but a milder fluctuation between fullness before feeding and softening after feeding will continue throughout your months or years of nursing. Anytime you miss a feeding or have a longer delay than usual between feedings, you will experience a notable fullness in your lactating breasts. As your breastfeeding relationship develops, you will look forward to nursing sessions as a way to ease your breasts' fullness as well as a way to nurture your baby.

◆ NIPPLE TENDERNESS

Many mothers worry that nipple tenderness automatically means something is wrong with the way their babies are nursing. While extremely painful nipples indicate that your baby is not latching on correctly or that some other problem needs to be remedied (such as an infection—see Chapter 8), a certain amount of nipple sensitivity or tenderness is common during the early days of breastfeeding. This is true even among mothers who are nursing successfully, especially if they are quite fair-skinned or live in areas with a dry climate. Usually, this sensitivity fades after the first few suckles on the breast and disappears completely after the first week or so. If you find that your nipples have become excessively raw, cracked, or are bleeding, try soothing them with colostrum or breastmilk, which can be expressed and spread over the nipples. An alternative treatment is to apply purified, medical-grade lanolin (available at your local pharmacy) after you feed the baby and expose the nipple to the air. Refer to Chapter 8 for more pointers and ask your pediatrician for advice. Keep in mind that preventing or treating nipple soreness involves working with your baby to make sure that he is latching on by taking as much of the areola into his wide-open mouth as possible and is not just sucking on the nipple. Rotating the positions you use when feeding your baby will also help.

◆ THE FIRST CHECKUP

While all of these signs and conditions are useful ways to monitor your baby's and your own breastfeeding progress, there is no substitute for that first visit to your child's pediatrician, no later than two or three days after your discharge from the hospital. By having your baby weighed, your breasts assessed, your breastfeeding observed, and your questions answered at this early stage, most potential breastfeeding problems can be prevented or corrected before they cause any lasting damage.

While human milk is the best, most nutritious food for babies, check with your pediatrician about whether you should supplement your baby with vitamin D. Your pediatrician is your best source for discussing all aspects of infant nutrition.

When to Call an Expert

WARNING SIGNS OF PROBLEMS IN BREASTFEEDING

Natural as the breastfeeding process is, problems can occasionally arise. When they do surface, they may grow worse very quickly and interfere with your milk production or your baby's ability to get the nutrition she needs. For this reason, it's vital to get help right away if you experience difficulty with breastfeeding at home or observe any of the symptoms listed below. Contact your baby's pediatrician, and don't stop asking for one-on-one guidance until you get the help you need.

1. **Your baby's nursing sessions are either very short or extremely long.** Breastfeeding sessions that are consistently briefer than about ten minutes during the first few months

may mean that your baby isn't getting enough milk and that not enough milk is being removed to stimulate your ongoing milk production. Sessions that last consistently longer than about fifty minutes may mean that your baby isn't receiving enough milk due to ineffective suckling or low milk production.

2. **Your baby still seems hungry after most feedings.** She may not be ingesting enough milk. Consult your pediatrician and have her weighed right away. Meanwhile, double-check her latch-on and position at the breast to try and increase the milk she is getting.

3. **Your newborn frequently misses nursing sessions or sleeps through the night.** Frequent feedings around the clock are a necessary part of breastfeeding a new baby. Your baby requires a feeding every few hours to gain sufficient weight to thrive. If your newborn sleeps longer than four hours a night, wake her up and encourage her to nurse.

4. **You don't hear frequent swallowing when your baby nurses after your milk supply has come in.** Your baby will probably swallow occasionally as she begins to nurse, more frequently as she continues a session, and less frequently again near the end. Swallowing is an excellent sign that she is actually ingesting milk, and its absence should prompt you to call her pediatrician at once. (Remember, though, that you may not be able to hear your baby swallowing when she is taking small sips of colostrum in the early days.)

5. **By two weeks of age, your baby is under her birthweight or hasn't started gaining at least five to seven ounces per week once your milk has come in.** Inadequate weight gain is one of the strongest indicators that a baby is not getting enough milk.

6. **After seven days, your baby has fewer than six wet diapers and four stools per day, her urine is dark yellow or specked with red, or her stools are still dark rather than yellow and loose.** If you or your pediatrician is concerned about your child's milk intake, you might want to keep a written record of your baby's wet diapers and bowel movements during the early days to be sure she is progressing properly. Most hospitals and lactation specialists can provide you with a special diary to use in recording your newborn's feedings and diaper changes, or you can use the one provided in the appendix.

7. **After five days, your milk hasn't come in or your breasts don't feel as though they're filling with milk.** If you feel this way, have your baby weighed by her pediatrician immediately. This is the most precise way to tell whether she is ingesting enough milk. You may also want to have your breasts examined.

8. **You experience severe breast engorgement.** Hard, painful breasts may prevent your baby from latching on correctly and discourage both of you from nursing. You may need to express milk manually or with an electric breast pump until your breasts have softened somewhat. Severe, unrelieved engorgement can decrease your milk supply.

9. **The fullness and hardness of your breasts don't decrease by the end of a feeding.** Your baby may not be drinking enough milk or may be suckling ineffectively.

10. **Severe nipple pain interferes with breastfeeding.** Your baby is probably not latching on correctly. If you have severe nipple pain or significant cracking of the nipples that makes it too painful to nurse, consult your physician or lactation specialist. They can check for the presence of infection of

the nipple or a breast infection such as mastitis (see Chapter 8) and help you with any problems with latching on. You may need to start breastfeeding on the less sore side or even use an electric breast pump until your nipples have healed. Your lactation specialist or La Leche volunteer can show you how to do this.

11. **After a week or two, you don't notice the sensations associated with your milk let-down reflex.** Though this may not indicate a problem at all, it could mean that your milk production is low. Ask your baby's pediatrician to evaluate her and observe your breastfeeding technique. Your local La Leche League volunteer or lactation specialist can help assess the situation too.

FINDING YOUR RHYTHM: ENJOYING LIFE AS A BREASTFEEDING MOTHER

"I loved those first few weeks with each of my babies," Diane, mother of three, reports. "Spending that time pretty much exclusively with each other, I felt like we had time to get the major bumps ironed out. Afterward, we understood each other better, and I could handle the little surprises or changes in our routine that happened as time went on." It's true that focusing on your baby for the first weeks at home adds to your confidence and your infant's ability to master the basics of his new environment. By the second or third month you will have become familiar with your baby's breastfeeding "personality"—whether he is an eager, lip-smacking nurser or a drowsy, dreamy type who needs to be wakened occasionally to finish a feeding. You can probably recognize his typical early signs of hunger (lip and tongue movements, rooting, waving fists, alert and eager looking-around) and put him to the breast before he begins his cry of hunger. His feedings will decrease in frequency but perhaps increase in length as he takes advantage of long, leisurely sessions that give him all the nutrients he needs. While no set number of breastfeeding sessions is "right" for every nursing baby, you will soon grow accustomed to the number that is right for your child. Throughout the months ahead, his demand for food will surge and decline as he experiences growth spurts or varying levels of physical activity. Your early observation and experience of his typical behavior (along with the information provided in Chapter 9 and the advice of your pediatrician) will help you understand when these changes are natural aspects of your child's development and when they require treatment or some other response.

Am I Spoiling Him?

BREASTFEEDING ON DEMAND

As relatives and friends observe your readiness to respond to your child's frequent demands for feedings, you may hear a comment or two about "spoiling" your child. This response to "breastfeeding on demand" results from widespread confusion between the act of meeting a baby's genuine needs and that of allowing an older child to indulge in self-defeating behavior. By feeding your baby whenever he shows hunger (even if that's every one or two hours), you are teaching him that his needs will be met and that his parents are listening to him. Responding to a baby's cues will not result in a spoiled child but rather a confident and trusting one. And since breastmilk is easier to digest than formula, it's normal for breastfed babies to want to eat more frequently than formula-fed babies.

◆ REJOINING THE OUTSIDE WORLD

When you and your baby have settled into a comfortable routine, you may feel the urge to rejoin the "outside" world—to introduce your baby to those you love and to interact with other adults yourself. This transition should not be difficult as long as you are getting the sleep and nutrition you need to sustain your milk production and keep your energy level up.

Breastfeeding a baby while resuming your "normal" life should become routine relatively quickly once you are comfortable with several breastfeeding positions and different nursing clothes. You will discover some great advantages of breastfeeding—how easy it is to pick up and go when there are no bottles to prepare and no pacifiers to search for. And life is much less expensive when you don't have to stock up on formula every week.

A blanket or sling can help you nurse discreetly in public.

Getting out and about with a breastfed baby is easier now that breastfeeding in public is becoming a common and accepted practice virtually everywhere across the country; plus a surge of state and federal legislation protects mothers' rights to breastfeed wherever they like.

Still you may encounter the occasional challenge to your new lifestyle. Critics may admonish you for nursing in public, ask you *when* you plan to wean your baby (even when he's just a couple of months old!), or suggest you offer the baby a bottle of formula if your milk doesn't let down readily when your baby wants to nurse. (Even after several months, glitches occur occasionally in your supply-and-demand relationship with your baby as he experiences a growth spurt, you go through a stressful period, or other life events occur.) You may find situations in which you just don't feel at all comfortable breastfeeding while others are present, especially in the early weeks as you and your baby are learning your new breastfeeding skills. In these cases, simply excuse yourself and go to another area to nurse, or express your breastmilk ahead of time and feed it to your baby in a bottle when you need to after the baby is three to four weeks old. (See Chapter 9 for tips on expressing and storing breastmilk.) You may wonder how you will adjust to working while continuing to breastfeed. (Reading Chapter 10 ahead of time can start you on the road to meeting this challenge.) You may be separated from your baby for longer periods, requiring you to provide one or more bottles of breastmilk to your infant's caregiver to use in your absence. Planning ahead, along with your solid base of breastfeeding experience, helps you adjust to whatever changes occur. Once you have committed yourself to nurturing your baby in the best way you can, little can stand in the way of a lasting and fulfilling breastfeeding relationship.

◆ **WHAT ABOUT BIRTH CONTROL?**

Once you have settled into life as a breastfeeding mother, you will no doubt enjoy renewing your relationship with your partner as well. One of the welcome advantages of exclusive round-the-clock breastfeeding (no water, juice, formula, solids, or other supplements for the baby) is that it significantly reduces the chance of your becoming pregnant again during the first six months because it delays the resumption of your menstrual periods. If your baby is less than six months old, your periods have not yet started again, *and* you are fully breastfeeding both day and night, you will *probably not* become pregnant even without the active use of contraceptive methods. At about six weeks postpartum, once your milk supply is firmly established, you can probably begin using contraceptives, but be sure to discuss the issue with your infant's pediatrician and your gynecologist first. As we pointed out in Chapter 5, no harmful effects on infants have been demonstrated when using hormonal contraceptives, but their use may diminish milk supply somewhat, especially during the early weeks of breastfeeding and when combined with other "stressors" such as a return to work or less-frequent breastfeeding. Birth-control pills with high doses of estrogen are more likely to decrease milk supply. Condoms, a diaphragm, or a cervical cap and spermicide may be considered as alternative choices for now (even if somewhat less effective), since these forms of birth control are unlikely to interfere with your milk supply.

Q & A
Can I Handle This?

Q: *I lose track of how often my baby has breastfed on a given day or how many wet diapers she's had. Also, I have a hard time telling the difference between a "snack" and a real feeding. Is it important to pay attention to this?*

A: Since breastfeeding involves no bottles with milk measured in visible ounces, it is important to monitor your baby's milk intake in other ways—particularly during the early weeks and months of life. The best way to make sure your baby is eating enough is to have her weight checked regularly—at every visit to the pediatrician and even between visits if your pediatrician recommends this. In the meantime, try keeping a breastfeeding log or diary to note each nursing session and wet diaper. There's no need to be obsessive about this, but spot-checking can be very reassuring as you establish your milk supply, and the information is useful to share with your pediatrician.

Q: *My mother-in-law did not nurse her children and feels very uncomfortable with my nursing. She's supportive in her way but wants to feed my two-week-old a bottle. Should I give in and let her do this?*

A: It's more important to establish and maintain your breastfeeding relationship with your infant right now than it is for your mother-in-law to feed her. Try suggesting other ways to bond with her grandchild, such as cuddling her between nursing sessions, taking her for a stroll, bathing her, or changing her diaper. Explain to her how important it is for you to breastfeed exclusively, point out the many advantages breastfeeding provides for your baby, and ask her to help you out by respecting your wishes in this area.

Q: *My baby is four weeks old, and already I feel like I'm suffering from extreme sleep deprivation. How can I breastfeed on demand and still get enough sleep?*

A: Some families find that keeping the baby in bed with them keeps parents' sleep disruption to a minimum, while others express concern that such practices may endanger the baby's health. (See page 107 for the AAP's recommendations regarding safe sleep habits for mother and baby.) An alternative to co-sleeping may be to keep your baby close by the bed in her own bassinet. With your baby beside you, you need only roll over, pick her up, and place her next to you to breastfeed. If your husband is willing to change the baby's diaper when necessary, you can fall back asleep once a nursing session is over. Also, try to develop the habit of sleeping during the day when the baby sleeps. Some sleep deprivation is always part of the process of early parenting, but breastfeeding certainly disrupts sleep less than getting up and preparing a bottle of formula. And soon your baby will sleep for longer intervals.

A HEALTHY FAMILY: BREASTFEEDING FOR LIFE

Two months had passed, but Ayiesha felt years older and wiser in terms of her experience as a breastfeeding mother. In eight eventful weeks, baby Sophie had become a happy new member of her active family, and breastfeeding had been fully integrated into the family's daily life. Ayiesha was happy to observe that her son, Jason, now took his sister's nursing more or less for granted, even if he did still tend to snuggle close to his mother during breastfeeding sessions. She enjoyed her husband's renewed appreciation for breastfeeding, as it made night feedings easier and saved them a small fortune in formula purchases, and she and Paul reveled in the ease with which they could just pick up and go with a breastfeeding baby.

Ayiesha would be returning to work in a few weeks, but she intended to keep breastfeeding for another year at least—expressing milk in her office and leaving bottled breastmilk for

Sophie's caregiver to feed her. Combining nursing with a job wouldn't always be easy, but it would certainly be worthwhile. Once again, with this second child, Ayiesha had seen what great advantages breastmilk offers to a growing baby. *If any more babies come along*, she told herself, picking up her alert, wide-eyed little daughter and hugging her, *they're going to be breastfed too.*

CHAPTER 7

Good Nutrition Helps

"All during my pregnancy, I was so worried about how the food I ate might affect my baby's development. It was a relief to know I could relax a little after he was born. Since I was already in the habit of eating well and limiting things like coffee and alcohol, I was able to enjoy all my favorite foods while breastfeeding, and my baby did just fine."

—Alice, 38, mother of Noah

"This baby's in very good shape," Dr. Fershing announced, handing two-month-old Lucas back to his mother, Louise. "He's gaining weight and obviously appears to be thriving. How about you?" he added.

"Great, overall," Louise said, cuddling her infant against her chest. "Lucas is a great baby, and we've gotten into a pretty good feeding and sleeping rhythm. The only things is, I'm still tired a lot of the time—even after I've had a nap and with my husband helping out at home. I don't know, maybe it's normal if you're a new mother. I just wish I had more energy."

"There may be other reasons why you are still feeling tired," the pediatrician pointed out. "Stress and the increased demands as a new mother could be factors. But it wouldn't hurt to look at your diet. Have you been eating well?"

Louise tried to remember. "I haven't been paying much attention," she admitted. "I guess I've been leaning pretty heavily on frozen foods and takeout. But I'm still taking a prenatal vitamin every day, like you told me to."

Dr. Fershing nodded. "That's good, but a vitamin won't give

you all the carbohydrates, proteins, and fats you need to keep up your energy. And you know, if your body starts to run low on nutrients, it will direct whatever's available toward producing your breastmilk. Your own reserves could get depleted, and that could make you feel a little sluggish."

"Do I need to be thinking about being on some kind of breast-feeding diet?" Louise asked.

"Not really," the pediatrician said in a reassuring tone. "You don't have to be on a special diet while you're breastfeeding. Like everyone else, the healthier you eat, the better you'll feel."

YOU ARE WHAT YOU EAT

Your own first months with your newborn have no doubt been an exhilarating experience for you both, but this period can also be tiring and even stressful. With round-the-clock infant care as your top priority and other aspects of life clamoring for attention, it's not always easy to pay attention to your own needs. Fortunately, your body has been preparing for breastfeeding since before childbirth without requiring any special diet or additional nutritional help other than a daily prenatal vitamin or a multi-vitamin/mineral supplement. You will both get all the nutrients you need as long as you eat a healthy diet that includes foods from each of the major food groups in more or less the correct amounts. This basic diet will provide you with all the calcium, iron, protein, and other vital components you need to meet your nutritional needs.

To many new mothers—particularly those who are eager to return to somewhere near their pre-pregnancy weight—the volume of food recommended in the pyramid looks like a lot. Keep in mind, though, that a serving as described here is not a plateful. One serving of breads and grains, for example, consists of one slice of bread or only half a bagel or a half cup of cooked rice. (For more detail on serving sizes, please see Appendix 4, "Dietary Guidelines" on page 251.) Since each group contains a wide vari-

Food Guide Pyramid

A GUIDE TO DAILY FOOD CHOICES

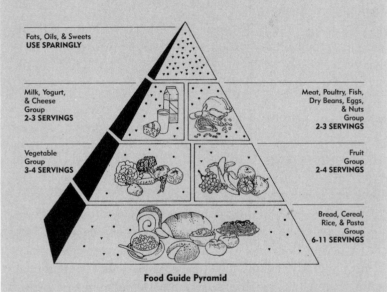

Fats, Oils, & Sweets
USE SPARINGLY

Milk, Yogurt,
& Cheese
Group
2-3 SERVINGS

Meat, Poultry, Fish,
Dry Beans, Eggs,
& Nuts
Group
2-3 SERVINGS

Vegetable
Group
3-4 SERVINGS

Fruit
Group
2-4 SERVINGS

Bread, Cereal,
Rice, & Pasta
Group
6-11 SERVINGS

Food Guide Pyramid

Use the Food Guide Pyramid to help you eat better every day. Start with plenty of breads, cereals, rice, and pasta; vegetables; and fruits. Add two to three servings from the milk group and two to three servings from the meat group. Each of these food groups provides some, but not all, of the nutrients you need. No one food group is more important than another—for good health you need them all. Go easy on the fats, oils, and sweets—the foods in the top of the pyramid. (For serving size information, please refer to Appendix 4, "Dietary Guidelines.")

Source: U.S. Department of Agriculture/U.S. Department of Health and Human Services ety of delicious foods, you should be able to find a number of dishes you enjoy. In the bread and grain group, for example, you can satisfy your daily requirement with corn tortillas (one per serving), hot cereal (half a cup per serving), pasta (half a cup per serving), or crackers (four per serving).

The most important concept to keep in mind is that your intake from the various food groups should be roughly proportionate to that suggested in the Food Guide Pyramid. The largest portion of your diet

Eating a balanced diet provides your body with the nutrients it needs for breastfeeding and good health.

should consist of complex carbohydrates, such as rice, pasta, whole-grain bread, and cereal. Vegetables should come in second. For snacks, try fresh fruits, vegetables, low-fat yogurt, or pretzels, for example, rather than rely on highly processed foods that are usually high in less healthy types of fat, oil, salt, or sugar. Your energy reserves will increase, and you will be eating the foods that are important for a healthy milk supply for your baby.

HOW A HEALTHY DIET HELPS
YOU BREASTFEED

For centuries, new mothers have been promised that certain foods or regimens will increase their milk production, stimulate their babies' development or speed their own return to their prepregnancy state. We now know that a normal, healthy diet is all

Don't Forget Water!

YOUR LIQUID INTAKE

Contrary to popular belief, no particular food or ingredient is guaranteed to increase your milk supply—but an inadequate supply of liquids can negatively affect your milk production and leave you feeling depleted. Whether you prefer water, milk, juice, or noncaffeinated sodas, keep something to drink nearby while you breastfeed, and make a habit of drinking enough to prevent becoming thirsty. All healthy adults are encouraged to drink between six and eight glasses of water per day. It is not recommended that you force fluids beyond your usual thirst. You should remember, however, that by the time you feel thirsty, you are likely to be mildly dehydrated. If your urine is dark yellow or you are constipated, you may not be getting enough fluid.

it really takes for a breastfeeding mother to maintain her milk supply and sustain both her baby's and her own health. Still, certain components of this normal diet are especially important when your body is producing milk.

◆ CALCIUM

Calcium, for example, is secreted from your body's stores (primarily from your bones) into your breastmilk to meet your baby's calcium needs. After you finish breastfeeding, your body must replenish the calcium that was used to produce your milk. Making sure you consume the recommended amount of calcium in a normal diet—1,000 milligrams daily for all women age eighteen to fifty and 1,300 milligrams for teenage mothers—may help to assure that your bones will remain strong after you have weaned your baby.

By consuming three servings of dairy products per day, as recommended for everyone in the Food Guide Pyramid, you should receive the calcium you need. If you dislike the taste of milk, you can get the calcium you need from cheese and yogurt. If you are allergic to dairy products, try calcium-fortified juice, tofu, or even turnip greens, broccoli, or dried beans. (Contrary to popular myth, it is not necessary to "drink milk to make milk.") If you do not routinely consume 1,000 milligrams of calcium in your diet, talk to your doctor or nutritionist about a dietary supplement of calcium. (Avoid supplements made from crushed oyster shells, though, because of concern about lead from these sources.) Consuming 1,000 milligrams of calcium daily— not only while breastfeeding but throughout life until you reach menopause—will decrease your risk of osteoporosis in later life.

◆ PROTEIN

Protein, another component of a normal diet that you should pay attention to while breastfeeding, can best be obtained through two or three servings of lean meat, poultry, or fish (about three ounces per serving); eggs (two to three per serving); peanut butter (a quarter cup per serving); nuts (half a cup per serving); or dried beans (1½ cups per serving). As always, it's best to vary your choices as much as possible, while keeping fat intake at moderate levels. Since peanuts are one of the foods most likely to cause an allergic response in both children and adults, be sure to monitor your baby's response when you eat foods containing peanuts, especially if there is a family history of food allergies.

◆ IRON

Iron helps breastfeeding mothers (and everyone else) maintain their energy level, so you may want to make extra sure you are including enough of this element in your diet. Lean meats and dark leafy green vegetables are good sources of iron. Other sources of iron include iron-fortified cereals and the dark meat in poultry and fish. (Certain types of fish and fish oils are also rich sources of DHA—docosahexaenoic acid—which is found in breastmilk and contributes to growth and development of an infant's brain and eyes.) Tea may interfere with absorption of iron or calcium, so you may want to avoid tea at the same time you consume dairy products or take your calcium or iron supplements.

◆ FOLIC ACID

Nursing mothers (along with all women of childbearing age) should get at least 400 micrograms of folate, or folic acid, daily to prevent birth defects in future children and ensure their baby's continued normal development. You can do this by consuming at least 2,000 calories daily and sticking to the higher number of servings of each food group recommended in the Food Guide Pyramid. Spinach and other green vegetables are excellent sources of folic acid, as are citrus fruits or juices, many kinds of beans, and meat or poultry liver. Breads, cereal, and grains are enriched with folate in the United States. All women in their reproductive years are encouraged to take a multivitamin supplement that provides 400 micrograms of folate daily.

In fact, it can't hurt to make sure you are getting all of the important vitamins and minerals by taking your daily prenatal vitamin or a daily multivitamin. Keep in mind, though, that these supplements are an *addition* to a healthy diet, not a replacement. The fact is, there is no replacement for a daily intake of fresh, vitamin-rich foods.

I Don't Eat Meat

SPECIAL DIETS

A special diet is often a healthy diet—in fact, you may maintain a particular diet for health reasons—but it still may not provide all the nutrients you and your baby need while breastfeeding. If your consumption of any major food group is substantially less than that recommended in the Food Guide Pyramid, consider how you will replace the missing elements in your diet *and* discuss your plans with your doctor or nutritionist. Breastfeeding women who do not eat meat, for example, must figure out how they will obtain sufficient protein for their babies and themselves.

As a vegetarian, you may already be familiar with ways to combine plant foods to provide adequately for your needs. Rice and beans eaten together provide more complete proteins than beans eaten alone. You can also obtain protein from eggs, nuts and nut butters, and meat substitutes. If you do not know all the healthy ways to compensate for lack of meat in your diet, consult a registered dietitian or nutritionist. Ask your pediatrician whether you should take a daily vitamin/mineral supplement containing such elements as iron, zinc, and vitamin B12. It is essential that strict vegans (who avoid all animal products in their diet) take a vitamin B12 supplement, since this nutrient comes only from animal sources. Keep in mind that you will also need to make sure you consume enough calories to maintain your health—usually between 2,200 and 2,500 per day if you are of average build. If you have any special concerns about your diet, your pediatrician may suggest you consult with a nutritionist.

WHAT TO AVOID: SUBSTANCES THAT MAY NEGATIVELY AFFECT YOUR BABY

Many women find the need to restrict or alter their diets during pregnancy difficult. It isn't easy for someone accustomed to five cups of coffee a day (or an alcoholic drink or two during dinner) to abruptly change her habits and adopt a healthier regimen. After nine months, however, the improvements to your diet and lifestyle may have become routine. If so, you're fortunate: Your new, healthier eating habits will help contribute to your baby's health and development. Still, now that your baby is born, it's natural to wonder whether it's all right to enjoy a cup of coffee with breakfast, a glass of wine with dinner, or even a cold pill when needed without worrying that doing so will harm your baby.

Fortunately, the mammary glands that produce your milk are able to provide your baby with highly nutritious milk even if your diet isn't perfect every day. As we discussed in Chapter 2, the mammary glands and milk-producing cells also help regulate how much of what you eat and drink actually reaches your baby through your breastmilk. Moderate consumption of coffee, tea, and caffeinated sodas is fine when you are breastfeeding. If you feel that your infant becomes more fussy or irritable when you consume excessive amounts of caffeine (usually greater than five caffeinated beverages per day), consider decreasing your intake.

◆ ALCOHOL

Alcohol passes through your milk to your baby, so it's best to avoid habitual use while breastfeeding. (Contrary to popular myth, drinking beer does not increase your milk supply.) If you choose to have an alcoholic drink, it's best to do so just after you nurse or express milk rather than before, and allow at least two hours per drink or two before your next breastfeeding or pumping session. That way, your body will have as much time as possible to rid itself of the alcohol before the next feeding and less will reach your infant. One alcoholic drink—the equivalent of a twelve-ounce beer, four-ounce glass of wine, or one ounce of hard liquor—will probably not harm your baby. However, there are concerns about long-term, repeated exposures of infants to alcohol via the mother's breastmilk, so moderation is definitely advised.

◆ CIGARETTES

Smoking cigarettes is not recommended for mothers who breastfeed. Nicotine, the addictive substance that you inhale when smoking cigarettes, passes through breastmilk to your baby. (Both nicotine and its by-products can be detected in the urine of babies whose mothers smoke and breastfeed.) If you do smoke, limit yourself to as few cigarettes a day as possible. Take your cigarette breaks immediately after a breastfeeding session.

It is also important to consider the effects of secondhand smoke on your baby. Inhaling smoke in this way has been shown to increase the risk of Sudden Infant Death Syndrome (SIDS) and is also related to an increased risk of respiratory illnesses such as coughs, asthma, and ear infection. To protect your baby from these effects, never smoke while holding or breastfeeding her, go outside of your home to smoke, and never smoke in your car. Residual smoke remains in your hair and on your clothing after you have had a cigarette, so your baby continues to smell and inhale it.

If you want to join a stop-smoking program or begin using nicotine patches or gum, discuss these plans with your doctor or pediatrician. Nicotine patches or gum should never be used by breastfeeding mothers who are still smoking, because the baby may develop toxic or harmful levels of nicotine in his system. If you stop smoking and use nicotine patches or gum, your baby will be exposed only to nicotine and not to the other by-products of tobacco, so this is preferable.

◆ RECREATIONAL DRUGS AND OVER-THE-COUNTER
   MEDICATIONS

In no case are recreational drugs advisable for breastfeeding
mothers, since their effect on infants may be harmful, lasting,
and, at the very least, highly unpredictable. Studies have shown
that SIDS is even more likely to occur among infants who co-
sleep with their parents when the parents indulge in recreational
drugs or alcohol. Indulging in drug use is clearly a bad idea for
any parent, and now is the best time to kick the habit if you have
not already done so.

Many new mothers wonder which over-the-counter medications are safe to take while breastfeeding. While most of these
products are not dangerous for your baby, it's always a good idea
to ask your pediatrician's advice before taking any medication.
Even when the product is approved, play it safe by taking each
dose just after you nurse rather than before. (For information on
prescription drugs, see Chapter 5.)

INFANT ALLERGIES AND
FOOD SENSITIVITIES

Human breastmilk typically does not cause allergic reactions in
breastfeeding infants, but mothers sometimes worry that their
babies may be allergic to something that they themselves are eating and passing into their breastmilk. In fact, only two or three
out of every one hundred babies who are exclusively breastfed
demonstrate an allergic reaction—and that's usually to the cow's
milk in their mother's diet. In this case, the infant may show signs
of severe colic, abdominal discomfort, a skin rash such as eczema
or hives, or may react with vomiting, severe diarrhea (often with
blood in the stool), or difficulty breathing that lasts up to several
hours after breastfeeding. If you note any of these symptoms,
contact your pediatrician right away. While rare—especially
among breastfeeding babies—milk allergies can be severe or fa-

tal. Most babies eventually outgrow allergy to cow's milk, although food allergies to other substances may be lifelong.

Breastfeeding exclusively for the first six months of life has been shown to significantly lessen the risk and severity of food allergies in families with a strong history of them. If your family has experienced severe food allergies, you might consider limiting your intake of milk and dairy products, fish, eggs, peanuts, and other nuts during pregnancy and while breastfeeding. Monitor your baby carefully for skin rashes, breathing problems, unusual stools, or other allergic symptoms, and be sure to tell your pediatrician about your family's medical history.

◆ FOOD SENSITIVITIES

A few mothers notice minor reactions to other foods in their diet. Some babies cry, fuss, or even nurse more often after their mother has eaten spicy or "gassy" foods (such as cabbage). These reactions differ from allergies in that they cause less-serious symptoms (no rashes or abnormal breathing) and almost always last less than twenty-four hours. If your baby reacts negatively every time you eat a certain type of food and you find this troubling, you can just avoid that particular food temporarily. If these symptoms continue on a daily basis and last for long periods, they may indicate colic rather than food sensitivity. Talk to your pediatrician about this possibility if eliminating various foods has no effect on your child's symptoms.

BACK IN SHAPE: A NATURAL APPROACH TO LOSING WEIGHT

A popular aspect of breastfeeding is the fact that nursing mothers regain their pre-pregnancy figures more efficiently than if they had opted to formula feed. The breastfeeding process makes use of the fat cells stored in the body during pregnancy. Every day

Q & A

Was It Something I Ate?

Q: *I've heard that colicky babies' symptoms can be eased if the mother stops drinking cow's milk. Is this true?*

A: In some cases, colicky symptoms do improve when the mother temporarily avoids cow's milk, even in cases when the infant is not allergic to the milk—perhaps because the infant's digestive system has not yet fully matured. If your baby exhibits such symptoms, discuss with his pediatrician the possibility of abstaining from cow's milk for two weeks, then starting back on milk and observing your infant's response. You will need to continue to have a source of calcium and vitamin D in your diet if you avoid milk and dairy foods.

Q: *Do the foods a mother eats affect the taste of her breastmilk?*

A: All the foods you eat will flavor your breastmilk. In fact, breastfed infants may be more accepting of new flavors and foods later because they have been exposed to lots of different flavors through breastmilk. Only in rare cases, however, do babies object to the taste. Even when infants do resist nursing, it is difficult to predict which tastes they will dislike. Generally, your baby may be most likely to enjoy the flavors of foods you enjoyed while pregnant. As with other food sensitivities, this is not an issue to worry about unless it frequently interferes with breastfeeding. In that case, eliminating the unpopular food is a simple solution.

that you breastfeed, your body contributes calories from these fat stores, in addition to the calories from your diet, toward your milk production. This is true even when you increase your diet by the three hundred to five hundred calories per day recommended to maintain your energy level and ensure adequate milk production. Keep in mind, though, that after an initial loss of about fifteen pounds immediately postpartum, this weight loss is *gradual*—occurring naturally at about one to two pounds per month for the first six months after childbirth and somewhat more slowly after that. In most cases, it takes about six to nine months (about the same length of time as your pregnancy) to lose the weight that pregnancy added to your figure.

In the meantime, it is much more important to focus on eating healthy foods than to worry about losing weight. Weight-loss methods such as liquid diets, weight-loss drugs, or severely cut-

Moderate exercise and a healthy diet can help you regain your pre-pregnancy shape.

ting calories can negatively affect your milk supply and your baby's health, so avoid them for now. If after six months of breastfeeding you find you need to lose more weight, you can restrict your caloric intake more aggressively after your child has begun to consume solid foods. For now, though, you can regain your figure at a natural, healthy pace by cutting out empty-calorie snacks, substituting skim milk for whole milk and broiled or boiled foods for fried ones, and exercising moderately.

EATING WELL FOR TWO

It was hard to believe that Lucas was already six months old. It seemed like yesterday when Louise first held him in her arms, and here he was able to sit up on Dr. Fershing's examination table, support himself on his pudgy little hands, and beam with pleasure at the doctor. "Congratulations, Louise, you have a fine, healthy young son," he said approvingly. "And you're looking healthier yourself these days."

"I feel better." Louise grinned. "Paying attention to what I eat has helped a lot—surprise, surprise. I guess it's normal to start getting your energy back after a few months have passed, but I think my healthier diet has helped. And it's a good thing."

"Why's that?" Dr. Fershing asked.

"Because Lucas is going to start crawling soon," Louise said, stroking her son's head. "And I'll need all the energy I can get."

CHAPTER 8

Common Problems:
Solutions and Treatments

*"The first couple of times you're faced with a baby who won't
eat, or sore breasts or whatever, you think, 'That's it, I'm
switching to formula.' Then, after a while, you find out that
most of these problems have easy answers. Once you get the
hang of breastfeeding, it really is a cinch."*

—Jackie, 24, mother of Shauna

"Rose? It's Vanessa. I'm sorry I called you so late at night...."

"Don't be silly. I'm only your best friend in the whole world,
who just happens to have been breastfeeding her own baby for
the last eight months! What's up?"

"I haven't been able to get Eli to breastfeed much since yesterday—not as much as he used to, anyway. He's been crying a lot
and acting like he wants to eat, but when I put him to the breast
he takes a swallow or two and turns away and starts crying."

"I can hear him crying. You sound pretty upset yourself."

"I am! I'm worried about him. He doesn't seem sick or have a
fever, but he's just not nursing enough."

"You may need to take him to see his pediatrician. But first let
me ask you a few questions. The way he turns away like that after starting to nurse, it sounds like the taste of your breastmilk
may have changed. Maybe he just doesn't like the new taste."

"You're kidding. How can it change like that?"

"Plenty of ways, I was told. Your body produces the breastmilk, so whatever affects your body may affect the composition
of the milk. Have you been eating any new foods lately?"

"Uh, no. Not that I can think of."

"Have you been taking any new medicines?"

"No. Everything's the same."

"How about exercise? Have you been working out a lot?"

"Well, yeah. I mean, he *is* five months old. I'm trying to get back in shape. I started working out at the gym a couple of weeks ago—with the weights and the step machine."

"How often do you work out?"

"Every day if I can, after Nathan gets home from work. I try to stay for about an hour."

Rose chuckled. "Well, that could be it! My doctor told me that strenuous exercise can create a buildup of lactic acid in your breastmilk. It doesn't hurt your baby, but it can change the taste of your milk. I bet if you back off a little on your exercise routine he'll be eating better again at his next nursing, but just to be safe, you should call your pediatrician in the morning if he continues to refuse to eat and is upset."

The natural process of breastfeeding fluctuates with the changes in your and your baby's moods, experiences, and physical state. Like most nursing mothers, you will soon grow accustomed to your own and your baby's typical responses to such changes and adjust your breastfeeding practices accordingly. You will discover over time that your milk flows more plentifully when you are nursing in a quiet place and feeling calm; that a certain way your baby fusses at the breast may mean he's coming down with something and should see his pediatrician; and that tenderness or soreness of your nipples can be cured by switching to a different nursing position.

At times, however, a new situation may surprise you. Your baby may suddenly appear uninterested in nursing or may frantically nuzzle your breast as though he can't get enough to eat. You may worry about passing on an illness that you've contracted. Or you may even find that your body has stopped producing breastmilk long before you are ready to wean. If you fear that such situations put your baby's health at risk or if they cause you physical pain, you will (and should) be especially eager to find solutions as quickly as possible. This chapter covers the most common stumbling blocks to successful breastfeeding. In many cases, the treatments and solutions offered here will be sufficient to help you overcome the problem. If not, however, seek the help of your child's pediatrician or family physician, lactation specialist, or La Leche League volunteer.

WHY DOES IT HURT? TREATING BREAST PAIN

"My baby, Sam, had a hard time latching on at first during breastfeeding," recalls Linda. "He always tried to suck just the nipple instead of taking the entire areola into his mouth. By the time we got home from the hospital, my nipples were really cracked and sore from our nursing sessions. I was actually ready to switch to formula because it hurt so much. Luckily, Sam's pediatrician was able to show me some new nursing positions when I brought him in for a checkup a couple of days later. She helped Sam latch on better, and this made breastfeeding much more comfortable for me. She also pointed out that the plastic-lined nursing pads I was wearing to soak up leaking milk tended to keep my nipples moist, which aggravated the irritation even more. Once I stopped using them and started using the new positions at home, I felt much better. I'm so glad I found a way to fix the problem instead of just giving up."

In Chapter 4, we examined the reasons why your baby's ability to properly latch on to the breast is the essential first step in learning to nurse successfully. In the days and weeks following childbirth, it is important to have your pediatrician or lactation specialist check to make sure that correct latching on has been achieved, since improper latching on can seriously decrease your baby's milk intake as well as your milk production. It can also cause painful cracks in your nipples that will make breastfeeding uncomfortable until they heal.

Many women find that their nipples are somewhat sensitive

Cracked nipples can be a result of improper latching on.

for the first few days, until they become used to breastfeeding. To prevent soreness, wash your breasts with warm water when bathing and avoid using soap, which can dry and irritate your nipples. If your nipples do become sore or even cracked, check again to be sure that your baby's lips and gums are on the areola as she nurses and not on the nipple. If possible, vary her position at each feeding. Avoid excessive moisture between feedings. If you are wearing plastic breast shells to treat inverted nipples, re-move them after thirty minutes, since these devices hold in mois-ture. Refrain from using plastic-lined nursing pads for the same reason. Gently pat your nipples dry after a feeding and then ap-ply colustrum, breastmilk, or medical-grade purified lanolin to sooth and heal them. (Creams and lotions generally will not help and may actually make the problem worse.) If these steps fail to solve the problem, ask your doctor, lactation specialist, or La Leche League volunteer for help. In most cases, nipple soreness is a temporary issue and should not stand in the way of successful breastfeeding.

◆ CLOGGED MILK DUCTS

Sometime during the course of breastfeeding, you may experience a sore breast or notice a small lump on your breast that may be red or irritated and hurts when you touch it. This lump may be the result of a clogged milk duct and should be dealt with immediately since it can lead to a breast infection. The best initial treatment for a clogged duct is to continue nursing, taking care to drain the breast as much as possible with each feeding. (If you suddenly stop breastfeeding, your breast will probably become engorged, which could make the condition worse and lead to an infection.) Before each feeding, gently massage the breast—beginning on the outside and working your way toward the nipple—paying particular attention to the firm area. Breastfeed as often and as long as possible, offering your baby the sore breast first if you can tolerate it, because your baby will nurse most vigorously on the first breast, thus draining it more effectively. Express milk from that breast after each feeding if your baby has not completely relieved breast fullness. Apply comfortably warm, wet towels on the affected breast several times a day (or take several warm baths or showers), gently massaging the area around the clogged duct down toward the nipple. If the lump on your breast remains for more than a few days, increases in size or redness, or you develop a fever or significant discomfort, make an appointment to see your doctor.

Keeping pressure off your breasts will help prevent clogged ducts. You can do this by wearing clothing that is not restrictive (avoid tight tops, bras, or underwire bras, switch to a larger bra size, or go without a bra for a while); by changing your nursing position so that your baby drains the milk from all areas of the breast equally; and by not sleeping on your stomach. If you notice dried milk plugging the openings in your nipples, wash them gently with warm water after each breastfeeding session. Continued difficulties with clogged ducts may signal a problem with your baby's latching on or with your nursing position. Arrange for a visit with your pediatrician or lactation specialist to correct these problems.

◆ ENGORGEMENT

Your breasts may ache at times when they become uncomfortably full, or engorged. Most mothers have experienced such fullness in their breasts, at one time or another as their bodies readjust to a baby's changing demands for breastmilk. A little fullness during the first few days after birth is normal, but excessive engorgement can be quite painful. Feeding frequently on demand helps prevent engorgement, but if your baby is nursing as often as she wants and is gaining weight, you may have to take extra measures to relieve the pressure on your breasts. You can, for example, soak a cloth in warm water and put it on your breasts or take a warm shower before feeding your baby. It may also help to express a small amount of milk before breastfeeding, either manually or with a breast pump (see Chapter 9). For severe engorgement, use a cool compress or ice pack between feedings to relieve discomfort and reduce swelling.

Discomfort due to engorgement may also be relieved by feeding your baby in more than one position. Try alternating sitting up, lying down, and using the football hold (see Chapter 4). Gently massage your breasts from under the arm and down toward the nipple to help reduce soreness and promote milk flow. If you have a forceful milk ejection that causes your baby to choke, try feeding her by lying down on your back with her lying on top of you. Take a break in the middle of a session to express a bit more if your baby starts to choke. While you do not want to take any medications without approval from your doctor, acetaminophen or ibuprofen may relieve pain and are safe to take occasionally during breastfeeding. Meanwhile, the best solution for engorgement is to keep breastfeeding. Soon your milk supply will better match your breastfeeding child's demand, and you will feel much more comfortable.

As strange as it might sound, one treatment for engorgement that many breastfeeding women have found effective involves the use of cabbage. Clean, refrigerated cabbage leaves can be either torn into smaller pieces, or left whole and applied directly to the breast. Whole leaves will conform to the shape of the breast if the large central vein is removed first. Held in place by the bra, the cabbage is left against the breast as desired or until it becomes warm and wilts. The wilted leaves can be replaced by fresh, cool ones. Either green or red cabbage can be used, but red cabbage is more likely to stain a bra or clothing. Many mothers experience an improvement in the pain and swelling of engorgement within hours after using the cabbage. There is limited clinical research on the use of cabbage for engorgement, and the exact way in which cabbage decreases breast swelling is unknown, but the treatment appears to be harmless. Regular application of cabbage has been used by some mothers to hasten the resolution of swelling or discomfort that occurs with weaning, especially when weaning occurs over a relatively brief time. For engorgement, cabbage should be used only until the swelling and pain begin to subside. Continued use may decrease the milk supply, i.e., cause your milk supply to "dry up."

◆ MASTITIS

When an area of the breast does not drain sufficiently, bacteria may begin to grow in that area and cause an infection, a condition called mastitis. Symptoms of mastitis include swelling, burning, redness, or pain, and you may have fever, flulike symptoms, or generalized aches. If you have any of these symptoms, let your doctor know at once. Treatment consists of warm compresses and antibiotics, along with frequent breastfeeding, rest, plenty of fluids, and pain medication. When your doctor prescribes antibiotics for mastitis, it is important to complete the entire prescription amount. Many mothers are concerned about the antibiotic being transmitted in the breastmilk and affecting the baby, so they either don't take the medicine or they stop earlier than recommended. The antibiotics given to treat mastitis do not generally cause any problems for the nursing infant, and failure to complete the course may increase your chance of developing another episode of the infection.

It's important to keep breastfeeding while you have mastitis, since frequent nursing helps drain your breasts and prevents the infection from spreading. Your baby will not be harmed by drinking your breastmilk. If it is too painful to have your baby nurse on the infected breast, move him to the other breast and open up both sides of your bra to let milk flow from the sore breast onto a towel or absorbent cloth. Frequently expressing milk from the affected breast with a breast pump will also help relieve the pressure and speed up the healing process.

CAN HE CATCH IT?
MINOR ILLNESSES AND INFECTIONS

Chances are that sometime during the course of breastfeeding you will develop a cold, the flu, a bacterial infection, or other routine illness. In such a situation, you may wonder if the baby will acquire the illness via breastfeeding. If you are nursing, your baby likely has already been exposed to the illness by the time you show any symptoms. It is best to keep breastfeeding, so that the antibodies your body has produced will pass through your milk to protect your baby. If you stop breastfeeding when cold or flu symptoms appear, you actually reduce your baby's protection and increase the chance of his getting sick or having a more severe illness if he does get sick. Even with more serious illnesses— such as gallbladder surgery or a severe infection—you can usually continue breastfeeding or, at most, interrupt feeding for only a brief time. If you are unsure whether a particular illness or infection affects breastfeeding, ask your pediatrician for advice.

One type of infection that may appear among nursing mothers or babies is a yeast or fungal infection. Thrush is especially common among women with diabetes and sometimes occurs after a mother or baby has completed a course of antibiotics. Signs of thrush in your baby include milky white spots or a coating on the inside of the mouth. Accompanying the spots in the mouth may be a diaper rash, also caused by the yeast. If the infection is on the mother's nipples, they may appear pink, shiny, oozy, crusty, or flaky, and she may experience a burning sensation in the nipples or breasts during or after nursing, even in the absence of other symptoms or signs of the infection.

To prevent thrush from occurring, keep your nipples clean and dry. Change your nursing pads when they become damp and wash your hands often. Be sure to boil or at least thoroughly wash with warm, soapy water anything that goes into your baby's mouth, including teething rings, pacifiers, artificial nipples, and toys. If you find signs of thrush in your baby's mouth or suspect that you may have a yeast infection of your breasts, contact your doctor and your baby's pediatrician. Always follow the course of treatment prescribed, and continue treatment until several days after the symptoms have improved or the infection may return. Do not rely solely on over-the-counter or home remedies, since these are not likely to completely clear up the infection. It is important for both you and your infant to be treated at the same time, even if only one of you has symptoms. This helps to prevent the infection from spreading back and forth between the two of you. Your doctor might advise you to throw away any breastmilk that you expressed and stored while you had thrush, because the yeast can contaminate your breastmilk and is not destroyed by freezing. While you are being treated, you can and should continue direct breastfeeding. Though thrush is easily passed back and forth between you and your child (as well as between sexual partners—a possible cause of your infection), stopping nursing will not cure the condition once it has developed.

Expert Help

WHEN TO CALL THE PEDIATRICIAN

Most routine problems that arise during breastfeeding can be easily prevented or quickly cured. There are times, however, when it is vital to have your child examined by his pediatrician without delay. Refusal to breastfeed may be a sign of illness that needs prompt attention. If your baby cannot or will not nurse for any reason, or you find you are having problems breastfeeding, make an appointment with his pediatrician right away. If your baby continues to feed poorly, your milk supply will begin to decline, so while your baby is being evaluated by his pediatrician, you may need to express your milk.

Other common infant behaviors or conditions that require *immediate* medical attention include extreme fussiness, fever, poor skin color, sleeping through feedings, coughing, or difficulty breathing. Repeated vomiting and reduced urination may also be danger signs. All of these findings are especially worrisome in a young infant.

WHY WON'T HE EAT?
COMMON FEEDING PROBLEMS

Feeding problems occur for a number of reasons, many of which vary according to age. In Chapter 4 we described very early impediments to feeding, such as a newborn's sleepiness or difficulty latching on. Most of these challenges can be met through proper breastfeeding instruction from a nurse or lactation specialist and the natural settling-in of a breastfeeding rhythm. It may come as a surprise, then, if your baby develops a resistance to feeding weeks or even months after you thought this was no longer a problem.

One thing to consider when this happens is whether the taste of your breastmilk has changed. Breastmilk taste can change for a number of reasons, including:

- a new food in your diet,
- a new medicine you are taking,
- a new pregnancy, which sometimes causes nursing babies to wean themselves a few weeks or months after the mother conceives,
- strenuous exercise, which can lead to a temporary buildup of lactic acid,
- a breast infection, such as mastitis,
- a change in the taste of your skin caused by using lotion, cream, or oil on your breasts.

Avoiding the new food, changing or stopping your medication if possible, exercising less strenuously, or refraining from applying oil or lotion to your breasts may be all that is necessary to encourage your baby to breastfeed at his normal rate again. If you have mastitis, seek treatment from your doctor right away and encourage your baby to breastfeed in order to drain your breasts. Once the infection has been treated and has passed, the taste of your breastmilk will return to normal. You may be able to help your baby adjust to the new taste of your breastmilk during pregnancy if you are persistent and patient and hold off on offering formula as an alternative.

If your baby starts to engage in frenzied short feedings that seem to signal frantic hunger, it may simply mean that your letdown reflex is occurring more slowly than she would like. If this is the case, try massaging your breast and expressing a little milk before you begin a feeding. This way, your milk will flow faster from the very beginning of the feeding and your baby will feel more satisfied.

If you do not believe that the taste of your breastmilk has been altered or that your let-down reflex is causing the problem, consider whether you are experiencing a high level of tension or stress. Such emotional discomfort can be communicated to your baby, preventing her from settling down to feed well. Of course, we cannot always eradicate stress from our lives, but for the moments preceding breastfeeding, do your best to put upsetting thoughts out of your mind. More-relaxed sessions will not only help your baby get more milk but may decrease your own stress level. Meanwhile, consider ways in which you might improve the general tenor of your day-to-day life.

It is also possible that your baby's own condition may be making it harder for her to breastfeed. Decreased interest in feeding— possibly accompanied by lethargy, fever, vomiting or diarrhea, cough, or difficulty breathing—may indicate an illness. Consult your pediatrician or family physician if your baby resists feeding or you have any concerns that your infant may be sick.

Illness in your infant may affect your baby's feeding pattern and desire to nurse, thus decreasing the amount of breastmilk she receives. If she has a cold, clogged nostrils may make it difficult for her to breathe while feeding, or an ear infection may make nursing painful. Clearing the infant's nasal passages with the use of a bulb syringe prior to feeding may help with temporary nasal congestion. Teething can cause gum pain when nursing. As pointed out above, thrush can make nursing painful and requires a pediatrician's attention.

Some babies take in a great deal of milk but then spit up what appears to be a large part of it after each feeding. Spitting up is a common reaction during or after feeding, and some babies spit up more easily than others. There is no need to be concerned, however, that your baby's spitting up is preventing her from obtaining enough milk. Spitting up (as well as hiccups) can be minimized by keeping your breastfeeding sessions as calm, quiet, and leisurely as possible. Avoid interruptions, sudden noises, bright lights, and other distractions. Try to hold your baby more upright during and right after feedings, and attempt to burp her after she finishes each breast. Don't jostle or play vigorously with her immediately after she has breastfed. If she vomits forcefully a number of times or if you notice blood or a dark green color when she vomits, call your pediatrician right away. Occasional small spit-ups or wet burps are generally more a laundry problem than a medical one. Fortunately, breastfed milk is less likely to smell sour or cause clothing to stain than infant formula.

◆ DEHYDRATION

As always, the best way to be sure your baby is getting enough milk is to monitor her physical condition, her weight gain, and the content of her diapers. It is very important to call your pediatrician if you notice that your child is not showing usual interest in feeding, she has a dry mouth or eyes, or she is producing fewer wet diapers than usual. These may be signs of dehydration. Severe dehydration, while uncommon in adequately breastfed infants, can be extremely dangerous or even life-threatening and is most likely to occur when a young baby refuses to feed or is experiencing frequent vomiting or diarrhea.

PROBLEM SOLVED

"Rose? It's Vanessa."

"Hi, Vanessa! How's Eli doing?"

"That's what I was calling about. I just wanted to thank you. His appetite has really shot up this week since I cut down my gym sessions to three half-hours a week. I guess he's trying to make up for lost time."

"Oh, great! So that *was* the reason, huh? I thought it might be. The same thing happened to me with my second child."

"Really? Well, yeah. I took him to Dr. Raines, of course, but he checked out fine. It really seemed to be a change in the taste of my breastmilk. Anyway, I have you to thank. Believe me, I never in a million years would have thought a strenuous exercise routine had anything to do with Eli's eating habits."

"Yeah, it takes experience, I guess. I'm glad you're both well."

"Both well and still breastfeeding. And the way Eli's enjoying his meals, it looks like it will be a while before we stop that."

CHAPTER 9

Breastfeeding Beyond Infancy

*"My daughter is eleven months old, and we don't plan to wean
any time in the near future. We are so in tune with each other,
thanks to the bonding of breastfeeding—and I can see that this
will make other areas of parenting, such as discipline, easier."*

—Elise, 25, mother of Sarah

In early spring, Jennifer was enjoying the gorgeous afternoon at
an outdoor café with her seven-month-old daughter, Maddie, her
sister-in-law, Liz, and her mother-in-law, Anne. Though Maddie
was her first child, Jennifer felt like an old hand at breastfeeding
by now, and she had no problem nursing Maddie as she chatted
with her relatives. "I've never had the garden salad here," she said
to Anne. "Do you know if they—ouch!"

Jennifer pulled back suddenly, looking down at her baby.

"What happened?" Liz asked.

"She bit me!" Jennifer said with a little laugh. "I think Maddie
has a tooth!"

Jennifer held Maddie up to see the first tiny white point protruding from her gums as Liz commented wryly, "That's the end
of the breastfeeding, I guess. I remember when my Robbie's first
teeth came in. I weaned him so fast he didn't know what hit him."

"Why?" Jennifer asked, giving Maddie a quick kiss on the top
of her head before she resumed nursing. "You can breastfeed after
your baby's teeth come in. Just because he has teeth doesn't mean
he doesn't still need to breastfeed."

"How long are you going to keep nursing?" Anne looked shocked. "I didn't breastfeed my babies at all."

"Well . . . that was a generation ago," Jennifer pointed out. "Before they found out how much better breastmilk is for babies than formula. A lot of people nurse their kids into the toddler years, you know." She looked down at Maddie, so content at the breast. "It's not just about nutrition," she added. "Every time Maddie is hungry and I offer her the breast, I'm showing her in a really basic way that I'm here when it counts and her needs will be met. Even when I'm at work and she gets her breastmilk from a cup, I think she gets the message that she can depend on Mom for the important things. I'd keep nursing through the first year just for that."

MORE IS BETTER

Jennifer's intuition concerning the value of breastfeeding beyond the early months of infancy is absolutely correct—yet, like her, you may face surprise or even disapproval as you continue breastfeeding beyond six months or into the second year. Our culture's past history of choosing formula-feeding over the breast has led to confusion over how long it is "normal" for a baby to nurse. Though most people know that mothers in many other countries routinely breastfeed their children into toddlerhood, the sight of an older baby nursing still takes some in the United States by surprise. Even some mothers who have observed the benefits of breastfeeding assume that the first tooth, the first step, or the first taste of solid food is a sign that the time for nursing is over.

Fortunately, this situation is changing. More families are learning of the American Academy of Pediatrics' recommendations that breastmilk remain an infant's sole source of nourishment for about the first six months and that breastfeeding continue along with the introduction of solid foods through *at least* the first birthday and beyond for as long as mutually desired by mother and baby. Just as your breastmilk provided the perfect feeding for

your newborn, so it continues to meet his nutritional, immunologic, and emotional needs as he grows. As he gets older, his relationship with you as a breastfeeding mother will develop too.
He will come to understand, in this quite compelling way, that
even as his world expands he can continue to count on you for
physical comfort and emotional support. What a wonderful les-
son this is for you and your little one to learn!

THE FIRST SIX MONTHS

It is wonderful to know you have triumphed over whatever uncertainties or challenges you experienced during the early weeks
of breastfeeding. Now that the two of you have settled into a
comfortable relationship, your baby has no doubt become a confident nurser, and your breastmilk supply and demand has stabi-
lized to some degree. You have probably grown accustomed to
her particular style of breastfeeding. You may also have experi-
mented with breastfeeding in public and have a good idea which
clothes, positions, and locations work best for you. As time
passes, you will find that breastfeeding is a perfectly natural and
almost automatic process as you take your child out with increasing frequency. You will be able to anticipate approximately when
your baby will want to nurse, respond quickly to her early signs
of hunger, and build in extra time for feedings when you are running errands or traveling by car. As you spend more time apart
from your child, you'll grow adept at expressing breastmilk ahead
of time so your baby can be cup- or bottle-fed in your absence.

◆ SUPPLY AND DEMAND: CHANGES IN YOUR
   BREASTFEEDING RHYTHM

Growing accustomed to your baby's breastfeeding habits
doesn't mean they will never change. As we pointed out in Chapter 6, feedings gradually become less frequent after your baby's
first few weeks, falling into a more regular schedule of feedings

throughout the day and night. Still, for a number of reasons, growing babies may abruptly increase or decrease their demands for feedings, resulting in an unexpected increase or decrease in the number and length of nursing sessions per day. An otherwise "regular" breastfeeder's sudden insistence on more feedings usually signals a growth spurt—a temporary increase in her rate of growth that requires an increase in calories. A marked increase in activity, such as learning to crawl or walk, may also cause your child to nurse more frequently as she burns up more calories or to nurse less frequently due to her interest in the new activity. Even stress or overactivity in your own life, which can cause your milk supply to decrease, may lead to her acting hungrier and wanting to feed more often.

The best way to respond to such increased demand is to breastfeed more frequently over the course of several days to increase your milk production and satisfy your baby's needs. (During this time, make sure you are getting enough rest and drinking adequate fluids.) Your baby will appreciate the extra feedings, and they will gradually taper off again as her growth rate evens out again, her activity level stabilizes, or your milk supply adjusts. Keep in mind, too, that if the appetite spurt occurs at around six months, your baby may be demonstrating her readiness to begin eating solid foods. As she begins to sample this extra

Breastfeeding should be your child's sole source of nourishment for about the first six months of life and should continue along with the introduction of solid foods for at least the first year.

nourishment, she will gradually depend less on your breastmilk to supply her with all the calories she needs.

◆ LOSS OF APPETITE

You may find at other times that your older baby has abruptly lost her appetite, feeding for short periods or refusing the breast altogether. In Chapter 8 we discussed reasons growing babies may lose interest in breastfeeding. In some cases, however, the reason for your baby's decrease in appetite won't be immediately apparent. If you have reviewed and discounted the possible causes for loss of appetite listed in Chapter 8 and have had your baby examined by his pediatrician and his health appears fine, you may simply need to exercise a little patience.

Meanwhile, resist the temptation (or others' urgings) to offer your baby formula or even a bottle of breastmilk as a solution to this problem. By using formula, you will decrease your level of milk production even more. By switching to a bottle, you may discourage your baby from returning to the breast when she is ready and able (usually after a couple of days). Better solutions include offering her your breast when she's sleepy and doesn't re-member to refuse it; trying new breastfeeding positions that may be more comfortable for her; feeding in a quiet, somewhat dark environment, without distractions from the stereo or television; and feeding her your expressed breastmilk with a spoon, eye-dropper, or cup if you are still concerned that she is not breast-feeding enough.

Eventually, your baby will probably regain her interest in nurs-ing. If not, it's possible that she is ready to wean or would be hap-pier with some solid foods in her diet. As always, it's best to follow her lead, providing her with the nutrition that best suits her age.

◆ IS SHE GROWING?

As your child grows, it's important to continue to monitor her weight to be sure she is getting the nutrition she needs. Refer to the standard growth charts on pages 164–67 for children from birth to thirty-six months to be sure she is continuing to grow at an acceptable rate, and talk to your pediatrician for assistance in interpreting your own child's growth.*

If your baby is older than three months and has recently stopped gaining or has even lost weight, consult your pediatrician, because babies at that age should still be gaining weight, even if the rate of gain has slowed a bit. An easily distracted, active, or impatient baby who is not feeding long enough in a session may need to breastfeed in quieter locations and switch breasts frequently in order to stay interested. If you have begun using a pacifier, baby swing, or other device to soothe your baby when she's fretful, try offering your breast instead—thus increasing her number of feeding opportunities. If she is teething (you'll notice her drooling more and perhaps sucking her fist) and thus enjoying her feedings less, make her feeding sessions shorter but more frequent, and give her a one-piece teething ring after each feeding. Again, these are simple solutions for most common problems that temporarily interfere with breastfeeding. If your baby's refusal to breastfeed continues, however, it is vital to have her examined by her pediatrician and to consult with a lactation specialist about maintaining your breastmilk supply in the meantime.

Though too-rapid weight gain is never a problem during the first few months of your baby's life (a younger baby should always be breastfed on cue), you may start to wonder if your plump older baby is breastfeeding too often. This might be the case for some babies if the breast is offered constantly, even when they have not signaled their hunger. If you do not believe that your

---

*Keep in mind that between ages three months and twelve months the average weight of breastfed babies is slightly lower than that of formula-fed babies. The standard growth curves used in the U.S., derived from analyzing growth data on predominantly formula-fed babies, overestimate caloric needs. Breastfed babies regulate their intake better than formula-fed babies, who have a greater likelihood of being overfed. We do not have standard growth curves available yet for babies who receive only breastmilk or, later, breastmilk with the addition of solids.

Your pediatrician will ensure that your baby is growing at a steady rate.

baby is hungry, consider exploring with your baby alternative ways for her to find stimulation or to comfort herself (such as bouncing on your knee, playing "peek-a-boo" with her sibling, or rocking in her father's arms). But don't worry too much about excessive weight gain during this first year. The fact is, most breast-fed babies regulate their intake of breastmilk to meet their needs quite well, and very few breastfed babies are seriously over-weight. Your baby will probably start to lose her excess fat as she becomes more physically active after six months of age.

◆ YOUR BABY'S TEETH

Your baby's first tooth will probably appear at around six months, though some babies are born with one or more teeth and others' teeth don't appear until almost a year old. As we saw

GROWTH CHARTS, AGE ZERO TO 36 MONTHS

Boys, birth to 36 months

LENGTH FOR AGE AND WEIGHT FOR AGE PERCENTILES

Source: Developed by the National Center for Health Statistics in collaboration with
        the National Center for Chronic Disease Prevention and Health Promotion (2001).
        http://www.cdc.gov/growthcharts
Reprinted by the American Academy of Pediatrics
The recommendations in this publication do not indicate an exclusive course of treatment or serve as a standard
of medical care. Variations, taking into account individual circumstances, may be appropriate.

Boys, birth to 36 months

HEAD CIRCUMFERENCE FOR AGE AND WEIGHT FOR LENGTH PERCENTILES

Source: Developed by the National Center for Health Statistics in collaboration with
the National Center for Chronic Disease Prevention and Health Promotion (2001).
http://www.cdc.gov/growthcharts
Reprinted by the American Academy of Pediatrics
The recommendations in this publication do not indicate an exclusive course of treatment or serve as a standard
of medical care. Variations, taking into account individual circumstances, may be appropriate.

Girls, birth to 36 months

LENGTH FOR AGE AND WEIGHT FOR AGE PERCENTILES

Source: Developed by the National Center for Health Statistics in collaboration with
the National Center for Chronic Disease Prevention and Health Promotion (2001).
http://www.cdc.gov/growthcharts
Reprinted by the American Academy of Pediatrics
The recommendations in this publication do not indicate an exclusive course of treatment or serve as a standard
of medical care. Variations, taking into account individual circumstances, may be appropriate.

Girls, birth to 36 months

HEAD CIRCUMFERENCE FOR AGE AND WEIGHT FOR LENGTH PERCENTILES

Source: Developed by the National Center for Health Statistics in collaboration with
the National Center for Chronic Disease Prevention and Health Promotion (2001).
http://www.cdc.gov/growthcharts
Reprinted by the American Academy of Pediatrics
The recommendations in this publication do not indicate an exclusive course of treatment or serve as a standard
of medical care. Variations, taking into account individual circumstances, may be appropriate.

with Liz at the beginning of this chapter, many mothers decide
that it's time to stop breastfeeding when they first notice a tooth.
Usually, this is because the baby has nipped the breast at the end
of a feeding session or because the mother fears she will be bitten. Yet many babies with teeth (or those who are teething) never
bite when breastfeeding. In fact, an actively nursing baby will not
bite, because her tongue covers her lower teeth. A baby who nips
the breast as he starts to pull away near the end of a feeding
can be taught to stop. It is a shame to allow this minor challenge
to get in the way of breastfeeding so early in your nursing
relationship.

If your baby has sprouted a tooth and you are concerned that
she may nip you as a feeding ends, keep your finger ready to
break the suction and remove your breast as soon as her rhythmic
suckling stops (and before she starts to drift off or feel playful). If

Nursing can continue successfully after your baby develops
teeth.

she has already bitten, say no firmly and then remove her from your breast. Try to keep this action as bland and matter-of-fact as possible: Too much anger or even amusement may interest her enough to make her want to repeat the experiment again. Once she realizes that biting means no more breast, she will learn to stifle the impulse. (Meanwhile, don't forget to offer her a one-piece teething ring when she is not nursing.)

Once your baby's teeth have begun to come in, it is important to keep in mind that even breastfeeding babies are sometimes susceptible to baby-bottle tooth decay (BBTD), a major cause of dental cavities in infants that can also cause serious damage to permanent teeth later on. Since BBTD results from teeth being covered with almost any liquid other than water for long periods, it most commonly occurs among babies who are put to bed with a bottle of formula or juice. While research shows that human

Clean your baby's teeth with a soft-bristled brush after breastfeeding to prevent tooth decay.

milk by itself does not promote tooth decay, breastfeeding infants who fall asleep while nursing and remain attached to the breast throughout the night with unswallowed milk in their mouths are also vulnerable to tooth decay. Beyond the first year, dental caries—tooth decay—can occur in toddlers who receive sugary liquids in a bottle or who are nursing and also eating foods with sugar and carbohydrates.

Your pediatrician will check your baby's teeth as part of the well-child visit during the first year of life and beyond. In the meantime, make a point of removing your breast from your baby's mouth once she has fallen asleep and wiping her gums and teeth with a piece of gauze or a damp cloth after feedings and before bedtime. To stimulate healthy gums and good oral hygiene, it is a good idea to wipe the gums at least once a day, beginning at birth, even before any teeth have erupted in your child's mouth. Once your child has several teeth, start using water and a soft-bristled, child-sized toothbrush for daily cleaning. Your pediatrician will advise you about when to begin using toothpaste with your child. Fluoridated toothpaste is not usually recommended until after age two, since babies tend to swallow it and can actually get too much fluoride. Some fluoride is good for strong, healthy teeth that are resistant to decay, but too much can cause a permanent, dark discoloration of the teeth.

WHEN MOMMY'S AWAY: FEEDING YOUR BABY EXPRESSED MILK

As you become more comfortable with the rhythms and routines of life with your baby, you will no doubt resume activities that were temporarily interrupted by early motherhood. You may need to return to work or want your baby's father or other caregivers to feed your child occasionally. In such cases, you can use a breast pump to express breastmilk that your baby's caregiver can then feed to him in a bottle or cup. This is preferable to offering your baby formula, since infant formula fails to provide him with all the nutrients of breastmilk, may decrease breastmilk's immune-enhancing benefits, puts some babies at risk of an allergic reaction, and may decrease your milk supply if you don't express your breastmilk.

An ideal time to introduce your baby to expressed breastmilk fed from a bottle is during his second month of life. Before about three or four weeks of age, use of a bottle may cause him to refuse the breast—a situation called *nipple confusion*. After age four weeks, he will be settled securely into his breastfeeding habit yet still be open to new feeding experiences. By occasionally letting him drink breastmilk from a bottle—even if you will not need to do so regularly until months later—you can teach him to switch easily from bottle to breast and back again. (This advance preparation is not absolutely necessary, however, since almost all breastfed babies can learn to adapt to alternative ways of being fed when the time comes. In most cases, they can adjust within about a week.)

◆ EXPRESSING MILK

Some women are apprehensive about the prospect of learning to express breastmilk. Like any skill, though, expressing milk gets easier each time you practice it. Milk can be expressed by hand, with a manual pump, or with a battery-operated or electric breast pump. Though hand-expressing can be challenging to learn for some women, it is the most convenient first choice, because there is no need for extra equipment (and, of course, it costs nothing). You might want to try this first during a regular breastfeeding, after you have already experienced a let-down reflex. You can express milk from the second breast immediately after a feeding with the first, or even during that first feeding if your partner or someone else can help you. Some women find that expressing milk when they wake up in the morning is easiest, since their milk is more abundant then.

To express by hand, first be sure that your hands and fingernails are clean by washing them with soap and water. (You might

To express milk by hand, press and release the areola between your thumb and fingers with a rhythmic motion.

even take a warm shower just before expressing, or place a clean, warm, moist towel over your breasts to help you relax and encourage the milk to let down.) Then massage your breast slowly, starting at the outer areas and working your way down toward the nipple. The massage should be gentle, never uncomfortable to your breasts or your skin.

Next, place a clean cup or jar beneath the nipple so that the milk will drip directly into it without touching your hands or your breast. Position your hand on the areola with the thumb above and two fingers below, about an inch behind the nipple (over the enlarged milk sinuses in the milk ducts). Press back toward your chest, then gently press the areola between your thumb and fingers and release with a rhythmic motion until the milk flows or squirts out. Rotate your thumb and fingers around the areola to get milk from several positions. Avoid squeezing the nipple or sliding down the breast, since this can cause bruising.

Transfer the milk into clean, covered containers for storage in the refrigerator or freezer (see more information on pages 175–77 on storing expressed breastmilk). If you don't collect any milk this time, try again later—but be aware that your let-down reflex may take a while to occur, and it may then take up to half an hour at first to sufficiently relieve both breasts. With practice, you will probably be able to shorten this time considerably and the amount of milk you collect will increase from perhaps an ounce per session to a full bottle or more.

◆ BREAST PUMPS

You may find it easier to express milk with the help of a breast pump. One of the commonly used manual pumps or hand pumps is the *cylinder type*, which consists of two cylinders, one inside the

You may find it easier to express milk with a hand-operated pump, like this trigger-type breast pump.

An electric breast pump that allows you to collect milk from both breasts simultaneously is best for mothers who express milk on a routine basis, especially if they have a hospitalized infant.

other. To express milk, you move the outer cylinder back and forth, creating a suction action. The milk collects in the inner cylinder (a plastic jar attached to the pump) that can be used as a bottle. Another type of hand-operated pump, called the *trigger type*, is shaped like a gun with a small jar for collecting the milk. This pump is operated by placing it against the nipple and pulling a trigger, which creates suction. The *bulb type* manual pump, which looks like an old-style bicycle horn, is not recommended, since the suction created is not usually effective and the device is hard to clean.

Small battery-operated or electric pumps are also available for women who express breastmilk only on an occasional basis. Full-time working mothers and those with premature, ill, or physically impaired babies who will be using a pump on a routine basis should use hospital-grade electric breast pumps. A pump with tubing and collection containers that allows you to express the milk from both breasts at the same time works best for this purpose. It's a good idea to talk with your physician or lactation specialist about what type and brand would be most appropriate before you buy. Many types of pumps can be rented instead of purchased, and there's no point in paying for a more expensive pump than you need.

Frozen Food

HOW TO STORE AND
PREPARE YOUR EXPRESSED MILK

Follow these safe storage and preparation tips to keep your expressed milk healthy for your baby:

- Wash your hands before expressing or handling your milk.

- Be sure to use only clean containers to store expressed milk. Try to use screw-cap bottles, hard plastic cups with tight caps, or special heavy nursing bags that can be used to feed your baby. *Do not use ordinary plastic storage bags or formula bottle bags, since these can easily split and leak.* Do not store breastmilk in ice-cube trays.

- Use sealed and chilled milk within twenty-four hours if possible. Discard all milk that has been refrigerated for more than seventy-two hours.

- Freeze milk if you do not plan to use it within twenty-four hours. Frozen milk is good for at least one month in a freezer attached to a refrigerator or for three to six months if kept in a zero-degree deep freezer. Store it at the back of the

Freeze bottles of expressed milk for later use. Milk is good for at least one month in freezers attached to refrigerators and three to six months in zero-degree deep freezers.

freezer, where the temperature is coldest. Be sure to label the milk with the date and time that you expressed it. Use the oldest milk first. Keep in mind that the fats in human milk begin to break down with storage, so using frozen breastmilk within three months is desirable.

- Freeze about two to four ounces of milk per container, to avoid wasting milk after you thaw it. You can always thaw an extra bag if needed.

- Do not add fresh milk to already frozen milk in a storage container.

- You may thaw milk in the refrigerator or by placing it in a bowl of warm water.

- Do not use microwave ovens to heat bottles, because they do not heat them evenly. Uneven heating can scald your baby or damage the milk. Bottles can also explode if left in the microwave too long. Excessive heat can destroy important proteins and vitamins in the milk.

- Milk thawed in the refrigerator must be used within twenty-four hours.

- Do not refreeze your milk.

- Do not save unfinished milk from a partially consumed bottle to use at another feeding.

◆ INTRODUCING THE BOTTLE

Once you have learned how to express your breastmilk, you will need to teach your baby to drink it from a bottle. Many mothers find that this works better if someone else offers the baby the bottle at first, somewhere other than where he usually breastfeeds. (That way, he will have none of the usual cues to start seeking out the breast). Clearly, this is an excellent time to enlist the aid of your baby's father or other loved one who has been eager to feed him, or perhaps to invite the baby's future caregiver to start establishing a feeding relationship with him.

During the first few attempts, have this person offer about half an ounce of breastmilk an hour or two after a regular feeding, when your baby is alert and motivated to try this new feeding method but not so hungry that he's upset and frantic. The adult should take care to keep a calm and reassuring manner; a smiling face and soothing voice will help your baby relax. It sometimes helps to drip a little breastmilk on the baby's lips or tongue at first to give him an idea of what you are doing. Then slowly and gently introduce the nipple into his mouth. Your baby should be allowed to explore the nipple with his mouth, not have it forced past his gums. Stop the attempt if he becomes frustrated or if more than ten minutes pass and he hasn't fed. It's better to end on a positive note and try again the next day than to create an association between this new method of feeding and feelings of frustration.

If after a few daily attempts he still refuses to drink from the container you've offered, try changing to a different kind of nipple or from a bottle to a cup. (If your baby uses a pacifier, he may prefer a similar nipple for bottle-feeding. Otherwise, you may have to experiment with several types of nipples until you find one he likes.) Some babies are picky about which feeding method they'll accept, but once they are introduced to one they like they adjust easily. Your baby may show a preference for a small medicine cup or a "sippie cup" rather than a bottle, even if he is very young. Be aware of your baby's cues and respond accordingly, but don't give up on any one type of feeding device until you've tried it for several days.

As your baby shows signs of accepting an alternate feeding method, start expressing more milk and occasionally offering the bottle or cup when he acts hungry between feedings. Finally, offer him (or have another adult give him) an occasional full, regular feeding with a cup or bottle at a time of day when eventually you expect to be absent. In this way, you can create a daily pattern that will be familiar to your baby by the time you need to implement it.

BREASTFEEDING FROM SIX TO TWELVE MONTHS

Breastfeeding, like many other aspects of parenting, is a gradual process of increasing independence and self-mastery on your baby's part, and a gradual "stepping-back" on yours. You may have already experienced the beginnings of this process during the first half-year of life as your baby learned to enjoy drinking expressed breastmilk from a bottle or cup and you began to go places without her now and then. Still, the two of you were closely tied to each other in a nutritional sense: Your child thrived on your breastmilk alone, which provided the nutrients she needed. During the second half of the year, your breastmilk will continue to provide the great majority of necessary nutrients as she starts to sample a variety of new foods. Though your baby will no doubt greatly enjoy the introduction of new tastes and textures in her life, her solid-food experiences are still just practice sessions for the future. It's important to make sure she continues getting enough breastmilk to meet her nutritional needs.

Opinions vary on how soon after six months to introduce foods along with breastmilk. Parents with food allergies are advised to wait until the child is at least six months of age and then to avoid foods that commonly cause allergic reactions (such as

This infant is showing signs of readiness for solid food.

cow's milk, dairy products, and foods made from peanuts or other nuts). If no allergies are present, simply observe your baby for indications that she is interested in trying new foods and then start to introduce them gradually, one by one. Signs that the older baby is ready for solids include sitting up with minimal support, showing good head control, trying to grab food off your plate, or turning her head to refuse food when she is not hungry. Your baby may be ready for solids if she continues to act hungry after breastfeeding. The loss of the tongue-thrusting reflex that causes food to be pushed out of her mouth is another indication that she's ready to expand her taste experience.

Since most breastfeeding babies' iron stores begin to diminish at about six months, iron-fortified infant cereal (such as rice cereal or oatmeal) is an excellent first solid food. Babies need only a few spoonfuls as they begin solids. Since these first foods are intended as complements to, not replacements for, the breastmilk you provide, it's best to offer them after a late-afternoon or evening feeding, when your milk supply is apt to be at its lowest and your baby may still be hungry. Mix the cereal with your breastmilk, water, or formula (if you've already introduced formula to your baby) until it is of thin consistency. As your baby gets used to the taste and texture, you can gradually make it thicker and increase the amount. When first starting infant cereal, check the label to make sure that the cereal is a single-ingredient product—i.e., rice cereal or oatmeal—and does not contain added fruit, milk or yogurt solids, or infant formula. This will decrease the likelihood of an allergic reaction with the initial cereal feedings. Some pediatricians recommend an iron supplement. If this is the case, be careful to give the exact dose prescribed by your doctor. Always store iron and vitamin preparations out of the reach of young children in the household, since overdoses can be toxic.

Once your child has grown accustomed to this new taste, gradually expand her choices with applesauce, pears, peaches, bananas, or other mashed or strained fruit, and such vegetables as cooked carrots, peas, and sweet potatoes. Later still, you can add

Q & A
What Changes Should I Look For?

Q: *I've been breastfeeding exclusively since my baby was born and assumed that I wouldn't get pregnant as long as that continued. Now that my baby is six months old, he's begun to eat a little cereal in addition to breastfeeding. Can I get pregnant now that my baby isn't breastfeeding exclusively?*

A: As we pointed out in Chapter 6, breastfeeding is a reliable form of contraception if you are exclusively breastfeeding, if your menstrual periods have not resumed, and if your baby is less than six months old. Once your baby is six months old and has begun sampling solid foods, breastfeeding is no longer a reliable form of birth control. If you do not want to become pregnant, you will need to consider what kind of contraception you will use. It's best to consult your gynecologist for advice on which types to use while breastfeeding, but in general, condoms, a diaphragm, a cervical cap, and spermicide are considered the most preferable forms of birth control for a breastfeeding mother, because they are least likely to interfere with milk supply. Low-dose birth-control pills should not have a significant impact on your milk supply when begun at this age.

Q: *I started introducing my nine-month-old to solid foods several months ago. Lately there has been some strange-looking red stringy stuff in his diaper. Should I take him to his pediatrician?*

A: As your baby experiences a variety of new foods, his bowel movements will look quite different from the yellowish, curdlike stool of an exclusively breastfed infant. It will begin to resemble and smell more like an adult's stool. You can expect occasional undigested or poorly digested elements to appear in his diaper. Babies don't really chew foods. They gum them and then swallow them, so when they start to eat small soft pieces of fruits and vegetables, you may see these in the stool. You can also expect a change in the frequency of stools after solids are added to the infant's diet. All of these are normal developments, but if you become concerned, call your child's pediatrician.

Q: *Is it okay to give my breastfeeding baby fruit juice every once in a while?*

A: After six months, you can offer your child small amounts of one hundred percent fruit juice fortified with vitamin C now and then—as long as the juice serves as an *addition to*, not a replacement for, her usual intake of breastmilk. Juice provides only a tiny fraction of the nutrients found in breastmilk; if your baby fills up on juice, she may actually become malnourished. For babies and toddlers, the American Academy of Pediatrics (AAP) recommends no more than four to six ounces of a vitamin C-fortified juice per day.

Q: *I taught my baby to drink from a cup at age nine months, and within a few weeks he had completely lost interest in breastfeeding. Did I do something wrong?*

A: Some babies do lose interest in breastfeeding between nine and twelve months of age, whether or not they learn to drink from a cup. Understand that he is not rejecting you; it's just the first sign of your child's growing independence. If you wish, you can continue to express your breastmilk for him to drink from a cup. His desire to feed himself "like a big boy" doesn't mean he has to give up the valuable nutrients you provide. He may still enjoy an early-morning or late-night breastfeeding session even after he has stopped nursing during the day.

such meats as turkey and chicken. Introduce only one new food at a time and wait several days before you add another new food, to make sure your child does not have a negative reaction. As you learn which foods your baby enjoys and which ones she clearly dislikes, your feeding relationship will grow beyond nursing to a more complex interaction—not a replacement for breastfeeding, certainly, but an interesting addition to it.

You may find that the number of breastfeedings will gradually decrease as her solid-food consumption increases. A baby who nursed every two to three hours during early infancy may enjoy three or four "meals" of breastmilk per day (along with several snacks) by her twelfth month. Unless you intend to wean her soon, be sure to continue breastfeeding whenever she desires to ensure your continuing milk supply. To ease breast discomfort, it may become necessary to express a small amount of milk manually on occasion, if her decreasing demand leaves you with an oversupply. Breast comfort is another reason why a gradual introduction of solid foods is advisable, since it allows your body time to adapt to changing demands. Over the span of several months, a readjustment in the supply-and-demand relationship can take place smoothly and painlessly.

BREASTFEEDING BEYOND THE FIRST YEAR

If you are still breastfeeding your child through his first birthday, you can congratulate yourself on having provided him with the best nutrition he could possibly receive. Now that he is consuming a wide variety of solid foods, your breastmilk has become somewhat less critical from a nutritional perspective. Some toddlers continue to consume a moderate amount of breastmilk (and thus the nutrients it contains), while others "graze" and ingest smaller quantities, getting most of their nutrition elsewhere. Certainly, there is no known point at which breastmilk becomes nutritionally negligible. What we do know is that as your child moves from babyhood toward toddlerhood, breastfeeding continues to act as a source of profound comfort and security, laying the groundwork for a confident, happy future. For this reason, as well as the continued nutritional and immunologic benefits of breast-feeding, the AAP advises mothers to continue nursing beyond the first year for as long as mutually desired by mother and child.

◆ STARTING THE JOURNEY TOWARD
SELF-MANAGEMENT

"I don't know what I'd do if Sam weren't still breastfeeding," one mother of a two-year-old said. "If he falls down on the play-ground and bumps his knee, he runs over to me, climbs into my lap, nurses for half a minute, and he's fine. When he's tense and on the verge of a complete tantrum, we take a breastfeeding break and in a minute he's relaxed instead of losing control. I know that some mothers wonder if breastfeeding at this age encourages an overly dependent relationship. But to me, it seems that Sam is learning to actively manage his emotions by soothing himself un-til he's at the point where he can deal with them. In the mean-time, he's gradually learning to cope by himself without running to me all the time. But after all, he's only two. I'm sure he'll wean himself when he's ready."

Many mothers do appreciate the power and practicality of breastfeeding to soothe a toddler's emotions, reassure him of their presence, and provide comfort in an often confusing world. Other women worry that continuing breastfeeding into toddler-hood prevents a child from learning to handle his emotions in more mature ways. The fact is, though, that toddlers need emo-tional reassurance frequently during the day. It is as valid and ac-ceptable for a toddler to breastfeed for comfort as it is for him to suck a pacifier or thumb.

◆ DEALING WITH OTHERS' OPINIONS

Our culture can sometimes project a somewhat limited view of acceptable breastfeeding practices; while nursing toddlers are becoming a more common sight, they still sometimes provoke comments and stares from uninformed adults. When deciding how long to breastfeed your child, a more valid yardstick than public opinion is your own child's approach to nursing and your own feelings about it. These feelings are no doubt being communicated to your child. Do you feel that he is dependent on the breast for comfort to the point that it interferes with his social growth (just as a toddler whose relationship with his blanket is so intense that he's unable to put it down to play with a friend)? Are you concerned that his continued nursing is causing other adults (such as a child-care provider, preschool teacher, or other important person in his life) to label him in negative ways? Are your own mixed feelings about breastfeeding a toddler interfering with your relationship with him—making you a reluctant and less supportive partner? If your answers to all of these questions are no, then there is no reason to hasten the weaning process.

My Turn!

NURSING YOUR TODDLER DURING PREGNANCY AND NEW MOTHERHOOD

Women who become pregnant while breastfeeding an older child often wonder whether they can continue nursing through pregnancy and after the new baby's birth. The answer is a qualified yes to both questions, depending on your medical history, your older baby's responses, your own feelings, and your milk supply. Breastfeeding mothers who have miscarried previously or who have a history of premature delivery should stay in touch with their obstetrician and report any uterine contractions, since the nipple stimulation of breastfeeding may increase your risk of delivering too soon. Most often there is no cause for great concern, but it's important to be sensitive to your body's signals. After the first few months of pregnancy, your milk supply will probably diminish somewhat, and the taste of your breastmilk may change as well. Either of these changes may cause your baby to refuse the breastmilk and eventually wean himself. You may initiate weaning yourself if you experience too much nipple tenderness or physical discomfort. If you and your older baby do continue breastfeeding, it is important to keep in mind that pregnancy and breastmilk production both require extra energy. Be sure to monitor your food intake as you prepare for childbirth and get plenty of rest.

Breastfeeding both your older child and your infant, called "tandem nursing," can in some cases ease your older child's adjustment to the new baby, address your own desire to maintain closeness with the older child, and even make child care easier in some cases as both children are fed and comforted on the breast. Again, though, tandem breastfeeding takes more energy than nursing a single child. Keep in mind that the new baby's breastfeeding needs are the most important at this time. Your infant urgently needs the colostrum (your milk composition will return to colostrum with the birth of your new child and will progress through the stages of milk as defined in Chapter 2) and immune protective benefits more than your older child. To ensure that your infant receives adequate breastmilk, breastfeed her before nursing your older child and allow her breastfeeding needs to take top priority. A one-year-old or toddler can make up for a decrease in breastmilk with nutritious solid foods. When taking care of a newborn or young infant, and older children as well, be sure to wash your hands frequently to prevent germs passing from one child to another.

Mothers who have chosen to continue breastfeeding their toddlers have found many creative ways of dealing with the surprise and uninformed disapproval they encounter among other adults. Many women teach their children a "code word" to use when they want to breastfeed (such as "Mimi" or "Nonny"), so that the matter remains private between the two of them. Some women then retire with their toddlers to a private place to breastfeed. On the other hand, others make a point of breastfeeding in public. "I breastfeed anywhere we go," says one mother of a toddler. "It can be done. The more this happens, the more acceptable breastfeeding will become."

Certainly, even in this country, the general attitude toward breastfeeding is gradually improving. Thanks to political activism by parents' groups in the 1990s, many states have enacted laws protecting a woman's right to breastfeed. Most of these laws state that it is a woman's right to breastfeed wherever she can legally be with her baby. In New York State, breastfeeding has been given the status of a civil right, meaning that women can take legal action against anyone who tries to prevent them from nursing. As more states create similar legislation, the act of breastfeeding will become more generally accepted, no matter what the age of the child. Federal legislation guarantees the right of breastfeeding mothers to nurse their babies anywhere on federal property where the mother and baby have the right to be. This is a good thing not only for mothers, who have so frequently been harassed simply for caring for their children, but for children, who benefit from all the nutrition, comfort, and love they receive.

WE'RE DOING FINE, THANKS: DECIDING WHAT'S BEST FOR YOUR CHILD

It was hard to believe, but Maddie was eighteen months old already, and Jennifer was proud to say she was still happily breastfeeding. Jennifer told her mother-in-law, Anne, that Maddie's sensitive, affectionate temperament would make longer-term breastfeeding likely. She was glad, because breastfeeding not only provided wonderful nutritional benefits for her child but kept the two of them in a lovely state of closeness. "I'll be a little sad to stop when the time comes," she admitted to Anne. Her mother-in-law looked surprised but said nothing. She had made a real effort to listen to Jennifer's opinions about breastfeeding. She knew that her daughter-in-law was doing what she felt was best, and that was all Anne could wish for her granddaughter. Certainly, her son agreed with his wife's decision to nurse until Maddie decided to wean herself.

Jennifer smiled to herself as she looked down at her daughter. Maybe breastfeeding had helped some other relationships in this family too. *Anyway, I wouldn't trade this closeness for anything,* she thought, as Maddie pulled away from the breast and grinned at her with a beautiful set of baby teeth (she hadn't clamped down on the breast in nearly a year!). Jennifer was so glad that she'd done her research and relied on her own instincts to decide what was best for her child, herself, and her family as a whole.

CHAPTER 10

When You and Your Baby Are Apart

"Expressing breastmilk at work is a nice way to feel that I am caring for my daughter, even when I am away from her."

—Alva, 45, mother of Celine

New motherhood was an amazing experience—both more joyful and busier than Betty had imagined while pregnant. By daughter Leslie's third month, Betty felt that she and her baby had begun to settle into a comfortable daily rhythm. However, they faced another major transition as Betty's maternity leave drew to an end and she prepared to return to work. Already, Betty had seen what an important role breastfeeding played in her daughter's health and in their relationship, and she was committed to providing her daughter with breastmilk through at least the first year if possible. Before she left her job, Betty and her boss had discussed how she could return as a nursing mother, and Betty knew that she was welcome to continue breastfeeding. Increasingly, though, she wondered whether she would really find the privacy, time, energy, and support necessary to maintain her milk supply. She knew she would be on her own for the most part in figuring out how to combine breastfeeding with high performance on the job.

Most women who hope to continue breastfeeding while working or attending school outside the home worry about how much support they will receive from their employer and co-workers or teachers and administration, and whether they will find the time and energy to accomplish their goal. The advantages are clear: By expressing milk at work or school, mothers feel more connected to their babies and are able to continue breastfeeding during nonworking hours. Companies find that breastfeeding women spend less time absent or distracted due to infant illnesses and are more satisfied employees who are likely to remain with the company. Still, the idea of combining work and breastfeeding is not a familiar one for many employers. If you intend to continue breastfeeding, it's necessary to prepare your employer, your baby, and yourself ahead of time, assemble a strong support team, and maintain optimism through whatever temporary challenges may arise.

HOW WILL I BREASTFEED AFTER I RETURN TO WORK?

Ideally, preparation for your return to work as a breastfeeding mother should begin long before you have your baby. While you are still pregnant, ask you supervisor or your company's human-resources department for information on the company's policies and history regarding *all* issues relating to a breastfeeding employee's return to work. This should include flexible work schedules, extended maternity leave, on-site child care (so the mother can make frequent short visits to breastfeed), bringing the baby to the office to breastfeed, and provisions for a private place and regular breaks for expressing milk for later use. In Minnesota, for example, companies are legally mandated to provide mothers with a place and time to breastfeed or express breastmilk for their babies. Elsewhere, an increasing number of employers voluntarily provide private rooms for breastfeeding mothers and even allow the baby to be brought to the work site to nurse. Larger corporations may provide one or more breast pumps on site for all their breastfeeding employees—selling or giving each such employee a personal kit that connects to the pump. In some cases, a lactation specialist is provided to answer questions and help employees learn how to use the pump and maintain their milk supply while back on the job. In short, you may be surprised at what options are available to you. Talk with other mothers at your company about what they have been able to arrange. If not much has been provided for breastfeeding workers in the past, perhaps you and any other concerned employees can volunteer to help establish these services.

In other cases, no provision at all has been made for mothers to breastfeed or to express milk for their babies while on the job. If this is your situation, you will need to talk with your supervisor about your needs. Such a discussion may be more successful if you come to the meeting with most of the solutions already figured out. Scout out a private, preferably quiet place where you would be able to breastfeed or use a breast pump to express milk. The ideal location for expressing milk would have a sink for washing hands and breast-pump parts, a comfortable chair with a table or desk to use for pumping, an electrical outlet, a refrigerator for storing the milk during the daytime, and a lock on the door. (You will also need a portable cooler with ice packs—the kind with a shoulder strap works best—to keep the breastmilk chilled as you carry it home.)

Of course, many women express milk or breastfeed at work in nonideal situations. If you have a private office you can install a half- or quarter-size compact refrigerator (available for sale or rent at relatively low cost) and wash your hands and pump parts in the ladies' room. (After work, take the pump parts home to be cleaned.) Many women obtain permission to install a table, chair, and refrigerator in a storage closet or other unused space, and they hang a *Privacy Please* sign on the doorknob if the door has no lock. If you do not have access to a refrigerator, you can store your milk in a small, portable cooler with ice packs. Be sure to place the milk in the refrigerator or freezer as soon as you return home.

You must also consider how you can schedule time for pump-

A private office with a door or a designated lactation room is ideal for mothers who wish to express milk at work.

ing or breastfeeding sessions during the workday. You'll probably need to express milk every three to four hours, around the times that your baby would normally breastfeed. Each session will last about fifteen to twenty minutes, though you should plan for slightly more time at first while you are adjusting to this new situation (the less time pressure you feel while pumping, the easier your milk expression is likely to be). Your traditional employee breaks and part of your lunchtime may provide you with the time you need. If not, you will have to ask for a little extra time, volunteering to make up that time in the morning or at the end of the day. If you foresee any potential scheduling problems or conflicts with other employees, come up with solutions ahead of time and enlist your co-workers' support. The idea is to demonstrate to the people who work with you that as a nursing mother, you will maintain your work productivity. As long as others are reassured about this, they will probably meet you halfway.

When you meet with your supervisor, lay out your plans simply and clearly. Describe any agreements you have made with co-workers about break times. If you know of other women who have expressed milk or breastfed at your company, refer to their experience to demonstrate that your solutions and concerns are sound. You might also provide information on the advantages of breastfeeding for mother, baby, and business obtained from the American Academy of Pediatrics (AAP) or La Leche League Websites (see "Breastfeeding Resources"). Most mothers find that their employers are willing to provide both a private space and use of break time.

Once you and your supervisor have worked out the logistics of your breastfeeding plan, write them down in memo form and ask your supervisor to initial it and give you a copy. This will prevent any confusion or conflicts when you return to work.

◆ AFTER YOUR BABY IS BORN

Even if you did not prepare for breastfeeding before your maternity leave, it is still possible to get ready before your return. Make an appointment with your supervisor to discuss the topics outlined above. During this discussion, reaffirm your desire to perform well at your job and point out that organizing a place and predictable times for milk expression will help you maintain work efficiency. If you meet with resistance, consider ways to schedule breastfeeding sessions on your own during lunch, scheduled coffee breaks, and before and after work—in your locked office, an unused room you have located, or even the ladies' lounge if necessary. Expressing milk in the ladies' room is the least desirable location, due to lack of privacy, concerns about sanitation, and aesthetically unpleasing surroundings, but many women have expressed milk there successfully if that is the only choice.

If you are threatened with the loss of your job because you are expressing milk, you can pursue several options. First discuss the situation with your supervisor, other superior, or someone from the human-resources department. At the same time, gather information and support from your physician, lactation specialists, or the La Leche League (see Chapter 3) and consider speaking with an experienced attorney. Unfortunately, in many states, employers are not required by law to support your nursing efforts in the workplace. But keep in mind that it's much better to try to settle any conflicts in a reasonable way rather than face the expense of a lawsuit. In many cases, your own positive, can-do attitude, bolstered by the knowledge that medical opinion supports your efforts, will deflect negative attitudes.

◆ **RETURNING TO SCHOOL**

Mothers who plan to attend school or college while continuing to breastfeed can use methods similar to those of working mothers. Discuss your intention to continue breastfeeding with your guidance counselor, a trusted teacher, the dean of women, or another appropriate member of the administration. Find out whether on-site child care is provided at your institution. (If it isn't and you are attending high school, ask your counselor whether there is another school in your area that does offer child care and other services for students with children. Your counselor may also be able to steer you toward parenting courses and La Leche League groups that can further support your efforts to breastfeed while attending school.) Ask for help in finding or creating a suitable place for milk expression—for you and any other breastfeeding students. Again, it is better to approach the administrator with a proposal already in mind than to expect others to make the effort to find space and time for you. If you can provide a clear, easy-to-implement breastfeeding plan, your transition to life as a mother–student should be a smooth one.

A Time for Everything

ALTERING YOUR SCHEDULE TO ACCOMMODATE YOUR BABY'S NEEDS

One way to successfully combine a job or school with breast-feeding is to change your schedule to accommodate nursing, if your personal circumstances permit. By extending your maternity leave, you will have more time to establish a breastfeeding routine. The longer you can stay with your baby full-time the better, so request as much time as possible. You might also explore the possibility of working from home one or two days per week—or even full-time—while you are still nursing. Perhaps you could start back to work or school part-time and gradually increase your hours as the weeks or months pass. (Mothers who work part-time are likely to breastfeed longer than those who work full-time.) Some breastfeeding women even share their jobs with another worker, giving them more time at home. Don't assume that your supervisor will refuse requests of this kind. Many employers understand that offering support to a breast-feeding employee offers long-term benefits to the company, raises morale (improves employee retention), and decreases retraining costs. You may discover that other women at your workplace may have already enjoyed such benefits. Unless you ask, you might miss out on just the arrangement that would work best for you and your child.

◆ SELECTING A CAREGIVER

Once you have a good idea what to expect from your employer, it's time to consider who will care for your baby while you work. If you can arrange for child care at or near your office, you may be able to breastfeed even after you return to your job by visiting your baby during breaks. Whether you plan to breastfeed during work hours or have the caregiver feed your breastmilk to your baby, be sure to select a caregiver or child-care program

What Would You Do If . . .

ISSUES TO DISCUSS WITH A POTENTIAL CAREGIVER

No parent wants to change caregivers once a relationship has been established. To ensure that your caregiver is the right choice for you and your baby—and that she will help you maintain your breastfeeding relationship with your child as you return to work—discuss the following issues with her ahead of time:

- Her willingness to feed your baby expressed breastmilk.
- How to handle and store your breastmilk.
- How your baby prefers to be held for a bottle-feeding.
- How to cope with resistance to the bottle.
- How to comfort your baby when he's upset.
- Whether she feels comfortable delaying a bottle-feeding if you'll arrive soon and can breastfeed.
- What to do if you're late picking up your baby.
- Your baby's eating, sleeping, elimination, and behavior patterns.

that supports breastfeeding and will follow your instructions for handling and feeding of your breastmilk. Discuss such topics as what to do about your baby's resistance to a cup or bottle, whether to delay a feeding if you are due to arrive soon, and so on (see box on page 195); be sure that your philosophy melds easily with the caregiver's intentions or the center's policies. At least once before you start back to work, leave your baby with the caregiver for a period of several hours that includes a feeding. In this way you can work out some of the kinks in the system that might otherwise prove discouraging later.

A MANAGEABLE COMBINATION: BREAST, PUMP, AND BOTTLE

Now that you have prepared your employer for your reentry into the workplace, it's time to prepare yourself and your baby. In Chapter 9 you learned how to use a manual or battery-operated pump to express milk for your occasional absences. For mothers who work regularly outside the home, however, a quality medium-sized or hospital-grade electric breast pump is much more efficient. A pump with connections that allow you to express milk from both breasts at the same time is best, since you will generally collect more milk in less time. This type of pump is also most helpful for maintaining a good milk supply. Electric breast pumps can be rented from your hospital or a medical-supply store, or you can buy one (see "Breastfeeding Resources"). Make sure that all parts of the pump that come into contact with your skin or breastmilk can be removed and cleaned. Otherwise, the pump can become a breeding ground for bacteria, and the milk will not be safe for your baby. Some mothers find that keeping a set of clean, duplicate parts at the office saves them a great deal of worry and comes in handy on days when they realize they forgot to wash out the pump attachments the night before.

You may not find it easy to use an electric breast pump at first, but with practice and help from your support network you will soon master the technique. The best time to practice is after a morning breastfeeding session, when you are likely to have a surplus of milk and your let-down reflex has already occurred. Beginning at least two weeks before you start back to work, if possible, try to express milk at least once each day, freezing the breastmilk for future use (see Chapter 9 for information on safely handling and storing breastmilk). Stockpile as much breastmilk as you can—at least enough to feed your baby on your first few days back at work and to allow for the unexpected (spills, missed pumping time at work, a sudden increase in your baby's consumption) during the first few weeks. Regularly pumping and freezing your surplus milk will not only keep your milk production high but will condition your body to respond to the pumping sensation with a milk-ejection reflex. Many mothers find that pumping more than once a day during this period adds greatly to their confidence as they prepare to return to work.

In Chapter 9 we explored ways to help your baby adjust to drinking breastmilk from a bottle or cup. Starting this process well before your return to work will help ease the transition for both of you, but your baby will probably adjust satisfactorily even if you have only one week to prepare. If you have already chosen a caregiver, these practice feedings would be an excellent way for the two of them to get to know each other. Just remember to wait until your baby is at least three to four weeks old, if at all possible, so that your milk supply is well established.

EXPRESSING BREASTMILK ON THE JOB

Readjusting to your previous work routine can be challenging enough without factoring in a breastfeeding schedule. Fortunately, you have taken the time to prepare your baby, your caregiver, your co-workers, and yourself for this new situation, so you are making the transition in the best possible way. Starting back to work in the middle of the workweek will make it easier for everyone to adjust to the change, since this will provide you with a two- or three-day trial period before you take on a full workweek. Plan ahead to take certain items to work with you each day. Many women get everything together the night before. You will need your pump, a cooler for transporting and perhaps storing breastmilk, and a lunch or snacks to help keep your energy up. You may also want to wear breast pads and pack a clean blouse or blazer in case of breastmilk leakage or spills.

On the first day back at work, check in with your supervisor; remind him about your agreement regarding your breastfeeding schedule and make sure that the space allocated for expressing milk is still available. (If possible, visit during your maternity leave to check on the space and to finalize any arrangements. This will ease your mind on that busy first day back.) When you begin your first pumping sessions, try to relax and keep your mind off the people waiting for you outside the room. Any stress could delay your let-down reflex or reduce your milk supply, delaying your return even more. Thinking about your baby—how comforted she will be as she drinks your breastmilk and how good for her your breastmilk is—may help you relax and start your milk flow. Some women find that looking at a photograph of their baby or even listening to a tape of her hunger cry works like a charm.

As you adjust to your new routine, you'll learn ways to integrate your pumping schedule into your day. This will become easier as your co-workers grow used to your brief absences one to three times per day and see that you can still be productive in spite of them. You will learn how to slip discreetly out of a meeting that has run long and is interfering with your pumping schedule—just as another co-worker might excuse himself to visit the rest room. You may even find how easy it can be to recover from or laugh at any snafus—a milk stain on a blouse or an interrupted pumping session—with the help of supportive and empathetic friends.

As you continue to express breastmilk at work, monitor how much you are producing. Diminished milk supply is a common problem for employed mothers and is most often the result of skipped pumping sessions or not pumping long enough. Also, pumping does not express as much milk as a baby can get from a breastfeeding session, if he is an effective nurser. To increase your supply, pump more frequently for at least ten minutes per session, even if your milk stops flowing before then. When at home with your baby, offer him the breast at least every two or three hours. If he sleeps through the night, consider waking him at your bedtime for an additional feeding. On weekends, breastfeed exclusively and nurse whenever he shows an interest. Once your milk production has increased again, maintain your supply by drinking an adequate amount of liquids, getting enough rest, and relaxing as much as possible during pumping sessions. Remember, cutting a session short to get back to work a few minutes earlier isn't worth the cost in terms of your long-term breastfeeding relationship with your baby. If these suggestions don't help after a few weeks, contact your pediatrician or lactation specialist for additional advice.

◆ ALTERING YOUR SCHEDULE

Many women have found that gradually adjusting their breastfeeding schedules at home reduces the need to pump breastmilk during work hours. Some babies are happy to increase their nighttime nursing to make up for one or two missed daytime feedings—eliminating the need for one pumping session per day. (This works especially well for mothers who are comfortable keeping their babies close to them at night—perhaps in a bassinet near their bed—so that they don't have to wake up completely to breastfeed.) Others find that, especially as their babies approach age six months, a feeding just before work, a bottle of expressed milk at lunchtime, and another feeding immediately after work is sufficient to get them through the day. Some women, who have well-established milk supplies, express more breastmilk on weekends than they normally do during the week to stock up on their supply. This means less pumping at work. As you experiment with variations on your original nursing rhythm, you will find your own best solution to the challenge of supply and demand. If you do not pump during the workday, you will notice a gradual decrease in your milk supply over time.

As your baby begins to sample solid foods and juices after age six months, you may find that you need to express milk at work less frequently. Some women choose to substitute one or more daily breastmilk feedings with formula or solids, eliminating the need for one or more pumping sessions at work. If so, plan to make this change gradually to avoid the risk of uncomfortable breast engorgement and an imbalance in your milk supply. Over the course of a week, pump less milk each time during the session to be eliminated, finally just pumping or hand-expressing enough milk to ease discomfort and prevent leaking. Continue to collect and store your breastmilk to freeze for possible future use. By the end of the week, you should have adjusted to the decreased number of daily pumpings.

By your child's first birthday, you will probably have stopped pumping at work altogether, simply breastfeeding when you are together and having his child-care provider offer him juice, formula, or milk when you aren't there. Looking back, you may consider the time you spent pumping surprisingly short—certainly worth the effort when you consider the many months of breastfeeding benefits your baby received as a result.

GETTING THE HOME SUPPORT YOU NEED

No one—especially a mother—lives in a vacuum, and you will find it easier to combine breastfeeding with work outside the home if you have the support of family, friends, and experts. In fact, lack of such support is one of the most frequently cited reasons that a woman might stop breastfeeding before her baby reaches the age of six months. Your adult partner can play a vital supportive role by helping your baby adapt to a bottle or cup as you prepare to return to work, by transporting her to and from the caregiver (or caring for your child himself when this is possible), by arranging for a quiet, uninterrupted "reunion time" for you and your baby at the end of the workday, and by reaffirming your decisions to return to work and to continue breastfeeding as you do so. Having your partner help with household responsibilities will allow you more time to either breastfeed at home or rest as you adjust to a busy schedule. Friends and relatives can lend a helpful ear, share their own related experiences and wisdom, and refer you to helpful groups, programs, and other information sources in your area. Your pediatrician, lactation specialist, and other breastfeeding experts can advise you on which breast pump is most appropriate for your needs, help you master the technique of pumping milk, and suggest ways to ease your baby's adjustment to a new feeding routine. Community breastfeeding support groups for working mothers can offer valuable management tips and reinforce your decision to keep nursing. If you have a caregiver who is supportive of your breastfeeding plan, you will find her help and encouragement invaluable. And don't

Q & A

Will I Be Able to Keep Nursing?

Q: *My boss and co-workers are very supportive of my efforts to continue breastfeeding. Oddly enough, though, my husband doesn't see the point of it. Now that we have a freezer full of expressed milk, he constantly suggests that I "just give the baby a bottle" instead of breastfeeding when we're at home. It's easy to get discouraged with the whole process when your family keeps telling you it's not worth the trouble. How can I get him to help?*

A: Your husband may not understand the role that nursing plays in maintaining milk production and may not fully appreciate the closeness and sense of security that breastfeeding promotes in your child. He may even be acting out of unacknowledged jealousy of the baby's central role in your life right now. Be supportive, but also remind him why you prefer to breastfeed, that expressed milk fed with a bottle is a welcome but less desirable substitute for the real thing, and that without frequent nursing your milk supply will soon disappear. Remind him how effectively nursing soothes your baby to sleep. Then spend some time and effort making him feel appreciated, so he feels like part of the family too.

Q: *I prepared carefully for my transition back to work, but in spite of all my efforts my six-month-old has completely lost interest in breastfeeding in the four weeks since I returned to my job. Is there anything I can do about this?*

A: Some babies—particularly those older than six months—do gradually lose interest in breastfeeding as they adapt to the bottle. Frequently this loss of interest is tied to a lower milk supply. To correct it, make a point of breastfeeding your baby frequently and always on demand—to comfort or soothe as well as nourish him. Breastfeed in a quiet, dimly lit place with few distractions, and consider increasing the number of night feedings. If he doesn't complete a breastfeeding session, pump the remaining milk from your breasts to increase your milk supply. Be aware, though, that some older babies simply wean themselves naturally at this point. If your baby has benefited from exclusive breastfeeding until now, congratulate yourself on providing him with the best possible nutrition for as long as he needed it.

forget to support yourself during this period by getting enough rest, drinking plenty of liquids, and taking time now and then for yourself.

WORK AND BREASTFEEDING: A HEALTHY ROUTINE

"Bye-bye, sweetie!" Betty said one last time as the family car pulled away from the airport curb with her husband and fourteen-month-old Leslie inside. It was Betty's first business trip since Leslie was born, and she felt a few tugs at the heartstrings even though she'd be gone only a few days. *At least I know Leslie will have fun while I'm gone,* she reminded herself as she carried her suitcase into the airport. She had worked hard last year to find a suitable caregiver for Leslie and didn't know what she would have done without Rebecca's support. Her husband had cleared his schedule to care for Leslie after work hours, and Betty's mother would be on call in case he needed help. Though Betty was still breast-feeding, she didn't need to worry about Leslie's nutrition in her absence either. Leslie had been eating solid foods for months and now happily drank other liquids from a cup. However, Betty had brought her manual breast pump along on this trip to pump for comfort and to keep up her milk supply.

Combining work with breastfeeding turned out to be easier than expected, Betty reflected as she joined the line at the boarding gate for her flight. She'd had her share of surprises (like the time her breasts started leaking in the middle of a company presentation), but even those were more funny memories now than sources of embarrassment. She had learned how to deal with such situations in a calm and professional manner. Looking back, the few months she'd spent expressing milk at the office seemed to go by in a blink of an eye, especially when viewed in the course of Leslie's breastfeeding over the past fourteen months. Expressing at work was certainly worth it in terms of the closeness she and her daughter had maintained in spite of their time apart.

One of the best "bonuses" of breastfeeding, Betty believed, was the way it enhanced her emotional relationship with her child. Many months of signaling and responding to each other's needs had increased their sensitivity to each other's feelings and helped them communicate effectively. Betty knew that when she returned from this business trip it was quite possible that Leslie would express resentment over her absence by acting out, retesting boundaries, or not wanting to nurse. On the other hand, she might climb right onto her mother's lap, relieved to find herself safe in her arms again. Both responses were normal, Betty realized, and experience had taught her that her own best plan was to respect her child's feelings, remain patient, and if necessary use her breast pump to maintain her milk supply until Leslie decided whether she wanted to resume nursing.

Betty took a deep breath, relieved to have a plan for this possible scenario. *Succeeding as an employed, breastfeeding mother may not be the easiest thing in the world,* she decided as she smiled at a couple passing by with their toddler, *but it sure gets easier with practice.* And the reward was a new confidence in her ability to manage her job and take care of her family too.

CHAPTER 11

The Father's Role

*"When we first brought Diana home from the hospital, I was
surprised at how much time my wife spent breastfeeding her.
At first, it was hard for me to get in any time with either
one of them. I guess I felt left out. But over time, I figured out
what stuff I was good at—like getting Diana to go to sleep
by holding her against my chest and singing 'Moon River' and
giving her a fun bath. Diana's nearly five now, and we still
spend a lot of time together on our own. I'm glad she was
breastfed and that I put in the effort."*

—Kevin, 38, father of Diana

Jacob's cry cut through the silence of the sleeping house, instantly waking his parents. "What time is it?" his dad, Ben, mumbled, glancing at the clock. "Four-thirty . . ."

"It's okay." Melissa, his wife, was already out of bed and stumbling toward the door. "Go back to sleep."

Ben fell back against the pillow, but it wasn't so easy to relax.
This was the second time tonight that Melissa had gotten up for
a feeding. Ben felt bad about her interrupted sleep—and, to be
honest, he wasn't crazy about spending half the night alone in
bed either. He guessed it was all part of the parenting package,
but he wished he could be more involved. *I never see them,* he
thought grumpily as he nestled deeper under the covers. *They're
together and I'm here by myself. When is it my turn?*

AND DADDY MAKES THREE

A great deal of attention has been paid to the new mother's emotional experience as she adjusts to the role of caregiver, but fathers, too, often feel overwhelmed by the elation, exhaustion, wonder, and concern that come with being a new parent. When the mother is breastfeeding, her partner may feel excluded at first as mother and infant focus on the rhythms of nursing, sleep, and play. This intense connection is a natural and important part of the newborn's life, providing a kind of bridge from prenatal to post-birth experience and laying the groundwork for a basic sense of security in later life. Yet studies have also shown that children whose fathers are involved in their lives from birth fare better cognitively, academically, and socially as they grow. Clearly, a child's healthiest growth springs from a secure attachment to *both* parents.

Making breastfeeding a priority gives both parents a chance to spend time together as a new family.

Did You Know . . .

FACTS FOR FATHERS ABOUT BREASTFEEDING

- Breastfeeding babies tend to be healthier than formula-fed babies—and there are no bottles, expensive cans of formula, or other equipment to deal with. You will save money you would have spent to purchase formula.

- Breastfeeding has been shown to reduce the risk of breast, ovarian, and endometrial cancer in a mother's later life and may reduce the risk of osteoporosis.

- Breastfeeding women use the weight (fat stores) they accumulated during pregnancy to produce breastmilk, so the more they breastfeed, the more likely they are to regain their pre-pregnancy figure.

- A mother's perception of the father's attitude toward breastfeeding is one of the greatest factors influencing her decision to breastfeed.

- Exclusive breastfeeding, with no supplemental formula or solid feedings, delays the mother's ovulation and works as a natural form of birth control for the first six months after childbirth, if the mother has not resumed her menstrual cycles and if her baby is continuing to breastfeed fully through the night.

- A breastfeeding mother whose partner supports her by taking care of household responsibilities is likely to be more successful and keep breastfeeding longer, enjoy family life more, and have more energy left over for her adult relationships.

- Babies' brain development depends on frequent verbal, physical, and emotional interaction with a familiar, loving caregiver. Babies need to be sung to, rocked, and played with as much as they need time breastfeeding.

- Eye contact between parent and infant is important for infant development. Mother and baby frequently make eye contact during breastfeeding. A father can maintain eye contact with his child while changing her diaper, giving her a bath, and playing with her.

- Growing children benefit from experiencing the different but complementary parenting styles of two different adults.

- The American Academy of Pediatrics recommends breastfeeding as the sole source of nutrition for infants for about the first six months; breastfeeding in combination with solid foods for the next six months; and continued breastfeeding thereafter for as long as mutually desired by mother and baby.

HOW CAN DAD HELP?
(AND WHAT'S IN IT FOR HIM?)

It is easy to say that fathers are important in the lives of their newborns and their partners, but it can be hard at times to see *how* to participate—especially during the early months. It may help to keep in mind that little things mean a great deal at this time: a word of encouragement for your partner as she adjusts to her new routine, an offer to help with the housework or care for the baby while she takes a nap, a confident defense when a friend or relative questions her decision to breastfeed on demand— these are small acts that let your partner know that you firmly

It's very rewarding for your partner to watch you breastfeed, and you will appreciate the encouragement and support.

support her decision to breastfeed and that you'll continue to support her. Many studies have shown the father's support to be the most important deciding factor in whether or not a woman chooses to initiate and continue breastfeeding. After all, you are the baby's other parent and perhaps your wife's closest friend. By seconding her decision to give your child the best possible nourishment, your actions can have a decisive and immediate impact on your baby's life.

One of the first steps you can take as the partner of a breastfeeding mother is to educate yourself regarding breastfeeding's many benefits. You are already doing that by reading this chapter (and, hopefully, the rest of this book). You might also ask your baby's pediatrician to discuss the advantages of breastmilk over formula and to give you an idea what to expect in practical terms during your baby's first few months of life. If at all possible, attend breastfeeding classes with your partner. By understanding how breastfeeding is accomplished, you can better help your partner after the birth as she learns such techniques as positioning your baby for proper latch-on. Learning about breastfeeding's advantages will also help you explain her choice to family or friends who don't understand or agree with this decision. Remember that many people still are not aware of the tremendous benefits of breastfeeding and have not been part of a breastfeeding relationship.

Immediately after birth you can support your wife's decision to begin breastfeeding by helping to make her comfortable in the delivery room. While in the hospital, you can take turns holding, rocking, and changing diapers so your wife can sleep between feedings. Also, you can support your mutual decision that the baby is not to receive a pacifier, bottle feedings, or sup-

Fathers can take an active role in their baby's care by bathing, changing, and burping the baby.

plemental formula without a clear medical reason. If your baby is unable to room-in continuously due to an illness, you can ask for a breast pump for your wife and help her assemble and use it.

Once you are all home from the hospital and family life has begun, your role as the partner of a breastfeeding mother will take on a new importance. As your baby's mother concentrates on establishing her breastfeeding routine, you can focus on keeping the household running efficiently and acting as a buffer for possible distractions to successful breastfeeding. If possible, take some time off work to prepare meals, keep up with the laundry, keep older children entertained, and otherwise allow mother and infant to concentrate on learning to breastfeed and getting the rest they need. Offer your partner food and drink while she's nursing, bring her pillows if she needs them to position the baby, and provide her with a

Babies love to snuggle after a feeding, a great opportunity for fathers to bond with their child and support the breastfeeding process.

book, telephone, diapers, or whatever else she likes to have near at hand. If you see that she's having trouble nursing—if her breasts hurt or she worries that the baby's not getting enough milk—use your own observations and insights to help her make adjustments in the feeding technique. If you see that she's still struggling but is reluctant to ask for help, remind her that successful breastfeeding is a priority for the whole family, encourage her to seek outside professional help, and tell her that you are there to assist in any way possible. Offer to call and schedule an appointment for her. She will appreciate your concern and steadfast support.

As you and your partner become more familiar with the routines of parenting, you can help with diaper changes, baths, and playtimes so your partner can sleep between feedings and perhaps enjoy a little time to herself. These interactions with your

Pitching In

TIPS FROM EXPERIENCED FATHERS

It's the little things. A word of encouragement or an offer to hold the baby can mean a lot to the mother and keep your home life more upbeat. Keep your eyes open for ways to keep both of your spirits up, such as bringing flowers home after work, telling your partner she looks beautiful when she's breastfeeding, and getting up first in the morning to take care of household chores so she can sleep.

Focus on the baby. Once the baby is born, your baby's mother may be preoccupied with learning new skills, relatives may offer conflicting advice, and your own work-and-parenting routine may feel overwhelming at times. It can be tempting to step back and let your partner handle new parenthood—but she will need your help in establishing breastfeeding. Think about your baby's needs and figure out how you can meet them most effectively.

Remember—this time will pass. At first, chances are you'll both feel tired or frustrated now and then. Talk ahead of time about what to do when you're tempted to snap at each other. A private joke, a kiss, or an offer to talk things through may defuse the situation. Keep in mind that what you are doing is important and you won't be new parents for long. Appreciate this amazing, unique period while it lasts.

Get to know your child. This is your baby too. Introduce him to your world, observe his responses, and begin enjoying your unique relationship.

newborn are excellent opportunities for you to create your own unique relationship with him. After feeding, a content baby is usually happy to snuggle up against Dad's chest for a nap or may be ready to play. Make the most of these moments—smiling and talking with your baby as you change his diaper, playfully splashing him in the bathtub if he enjoys getting splashed, holding and rocking him when he cries, and making up fun little games that he plays only with you. Babies also love to be part of such "grown-up" activities as taking a walk outside and "reading" books and magazines. As your child regularly experiences these times with you, he will understand that daddies aren't just mommy substitutes.

◆ COMBINING WORK AND FAMILY LIFE

Work schedules pose additional challenges to both parents of a breastfeeding child. If you work outside the home during the early months of parenthood, you will need to monitor your energy supply as carefully as your partner does. Try not to extend your work hours, take on extra projects, or travel much during this period if possible. If you find that you or your partner are feeling seriously sleep-deprived, discuss ways to reallocate parenting time so you both can have the time for sleep and relaxation that you need.

If and when your child's mother begins working

Your partner can help you by playing with or carrying the baby, assisting in finding a caregiver, and washing and preparing breast pumps for use.

outside the home, she will need the same consideration from you. Adjusting to her new responsibilities can be daunting at first as she meets such challenges as learning how to use a breast pump, storing breastmilk for future use, arranging for child care, and expressing milk on the job. You may be able to make this process easier in one of many ways—such as helping locate a suitable caregiver, packing the baby's bag before work each morning, preparing the breast pump at night for the next day's use, and making sure mother and baby enjoy an undisturbed "re-union feeding" at the end of each workday. You may also consider taking your child, when feasible, to the mother's workplace for a midday feeding. Keep in mind, too, that your wife may be more tired than usual as she learns to combine motherhood with a job. Make allowances for her limited reserves and work to keep the lines of communication open.

Of course, fathers can get tired and just plain discouraged, too, and at these times it helps to have a few people in mind who know how to help you relax and let off steam. Ideally, you will enjoy the support of male friends who also participated a great deal in raising their breastfed babies. Such experienced dads can offer solutions for problems, sympathy when things get tough, and suggestions on dealing with the unsought advice and criti-cism that some new parents receive. If you don't know any fa-thers who have played an active role in the lives of their children, contact your local La Leche League (see Chapter 3) for informa-tion on couples meetings. Finally, don't forget your female friends or associates at work, who can empathize with many as-pects of parenting life and offer insights about situations that con-cern you. Whomever you choose to talk to, make sure you do take the time to talk. Becoming a parent is an enormous transi-tion for every couple. Sharing both the highs and the lows with an empathetic friend will enhance and deepen your experience.

Q & A
Can I Do Something?

Q: *My wife believes strongly in breastfeeding on demand, but my parents think she's spoiling our three-week-old by nursing her every hour or even more frequently. They tell me that at this rate our child will never learn responsibility and self-control and that she'll grow up expecting to boss us around. Who's right—my wife or my parents? And how do I keep them all happy?*

A: Your parents' response to breastfeeding on demand is quite common but inappropriate, as was discussed in Chapter 6. A three-week-old baby is incapable of being spoiled and can only benefit from learning that her needs will consistently be met. You may not be able to change your parents' view, but it is important to express to them that you agree with the mother's decision to breastfeed whenever her child wishes. Your wife will appreciate your support and the fact that you and she are united in your decisions. By backing her up, you are creating a powerful parenting team that will serve the family well in the years to come. Chances are that eventually your parents will see that both of you made the right decision.

Q: *Our baby boy, Henry, is eight weeks old and has not yet slept through an entire night. My wife is exhausted, so lately I've been trying to give her a break by getting up to play with Henry for a while before she breastfeeds. Unfortunately, Henry just keeps crying the entire time, louder and louder, and my wife gets up and takes the baby. Is there some way I can make him happy so my wife can sleep?*

A: Your baby's cries are his way of telling you that he's hungry and needs to be fed. By responding to his needs, you increase his trust and attachment to you, thus laying the groundwork for healthy growth throughout his childhood. Tired as your wife might be, it's important for her to nurse your baby when he communicates his need. You can make night feedings easier by carrying the baby to her, letting her nurse while still in bed and half asleep, and then changing his diaper and helping him get back to sleep. Consider keeping your baby close by in a cradle or crib next to the bed so your wife doesn't have to get up to get him. Many couples assign the "day shift" to one parent and the "night shift" to the other—so that, for example, the wife tends to the baby at night, but after the first morning feeding, the husband gets up with him and takes care of his needs as much as possible during the day between feedings. Soon, feedings will decrease in frequency and your son will sleep for longer intervals. Meanwhile, your wife and child will be grateful for your help.

Q: *My wife and I separated during her pregnancy and she has custody of the baby. I would like to set up a visitation schedule with him. Is this possible with a breastfeeding infant?*

A: You are off to an excellent start as a parent by recognizing your child's need to breastfeed as a top priority at this time. Ideally, you will be able to work with the baby's mother to create a visitation schedule that allows for this need, rather than relying on a court-mandated arrangement that might be less favorable. The best visitation schedule starts with the length and frequency of separations from the mother that your baby already experiences, and gradually lengthens as time passes. If the mother doesn't work outside the home and breastfeeds on demand, you will need to begin with frequent, brief visits (perhaps visiting the child for an hour before work, during lunch, or after work on appointed days, preferably in the mother's home). If he is accustomed to longer separations with a caregiver, you can take the caregiver's place for the same length of time. As you increase the number and length of your visits with your child, discuss with his mother the possibility of using a bottle to feed him breastmilk she has expressed with a pump or by hand—and keep in mind that you will be able to feed him other foods after he is six months old. Once you have reached this stage and feedings are spaced apart more, it becomes easier for you to go out with your child for a brief time. Eventually, he will be able to happily stay overnight and on weekends with you.

BREASTFEEDING AND SEXUALITY

I'd heard all the jokes about what a new baby does to your sex life, a father wrote, *but when it happened to us, I felt like our marriage had been hit with a truck. All of a sudden, my wife didn't want to be touched anymore—ever! That was a hard part of adjusting to parenthood, but now we're back the way we were. Actually, I'd say our relationship is even more satisfying now than it was before our daughter was born.*

It really shouldn't be surprising that the experience of childbirth, a significant amount of sleep deprivation, and a radically new family structure can create some very strong shock waves in a couple's marital relationship, but many parents are startled by the swings in their feelings about each other and their desire for sexual contact. Complicating things more is the fact that mothers' and fathers' experiences differ in such important ways at first—with mothers in almost constant physical contact with their babies while fathers look on, desiring more closeness. At the end of the day, a new mother may have had so much "touching" that sex is the last thing on her mind, while a father may feel especially in need of some physical sign of her affection.

This is not always the case, of course. Some breastfeeding mothers (and their partners) experience less sexual desire during certain phases of parenthood, while others experience more. If you and your partner find that the intimacy of the breastfeeding period enhances your sexual life, or if you feel freed by the natu-

Pillow Talk

HOW DO YOU FEEL ABOUT BREASTFEEDING?

In a recent study, pregnant women were asked to predict what their partners' attitudes toward breastfeeding would be. Surprisingly, their responses were highly inaccurate (hardly better than random guessing). Most believed that their partners were far more negative about breastfeeding than they actually were. For this reason, it's important to share your feelings about breastfeeding and new parenthood with your partner whenever possible. Such conversations can help preserve the intimacy of your relationship during the physically challenging early months, while also supporting your wife in her breastfeeding efforts at a time when every encouraging word helps. If you love the sight of her breastfeeding your baby, tell her how it makes you feel. If you consider her lush, nursing mother's figure just as sexy, let her know. Share with her your pride in her commitment to breastfeeding as she breastfeeds in public and makes herself available to satisfy your child's hunger at all times. Such words of support and affirmation can act as a highly effective aphrodisiac for many new mothers (if not now, then later) and may improve your marriage even as they ensure your child's continued good health.

ral birth-control benefits of exclusive breastfeeding during the first six months, take full advantage of it. If, on the other hand, your desires conflict, try to take the long view. Remember that this stage will pass and focus on keeping the lines of communication open in the meantime. Your partner may respond more positively to kisses, an occasional nuzzle, or a back rub rather than to more intense physical contact. Sincere compliments can mean a lot to a new mother, who may feel less "put together" than she's used to and may feel a little self-conscious about her postpartum shape. Some men find that they like the larger breasts that result from breastfeeding. (Be aware that breastmilk can let-down during orgasm, causing some leakage. There's no need to worry about this "spilled milk," however. There will be plenty of breastmilk left for the baby.)

A recent study showed that most couples resume intercourse at about seven weeks postpartum, though breastfeeding couples' sexual activity tends to resume more gradually than that of bottle-feeding couples throughout the first year. By taking into account this typical pattern of sexual activity and understanding that it's a normal part of the transition from pregnancy to life as a family, you may be able to relax enough during this temporary glitch in your sex life to enjoy the wonderful changes that are happening in your family.

I'LL GET HIM. YOU SLEEP: CREATING A PARENTING TEAM

"What time is it?" Ben looked at the clock. "Four in the morning," he mumbled. "Why am I not surprised?" He rolled over in bed to see if Melissa was awake, but she had already lifted baby Jacob from his cradle and tucked him next to her in bed for a drowsy nursing session. *Putting that cradle in our room was one of the best ideas we've had*, Ben thought as he rolled over to go back to sleep. Another good idea was discussing with Melissa how they would divide parenting duties, and planning their schedules accordingly.

Now Ben could sleep guilt-free, knowing that he would take Jacob after his early-morning feeding so that Melissa could sleep a little longer. Ben had found that he actually enjoyed making breakfast and straightening the house first thing every day, while Jacob peeked out from the carrier on his chest. Before leaving for work, Ben made sure that Melissa had the baby supplies she needed for the day. When he got home in the evenings, he cuddled and held Jacob so Melissa could have time for herself or take a nap.

Far from feeling separated from his small family, Ben had begun to see himself as a valuable part of the parenting team. He and Jacob had found that they enjoyed listening to music and reading books together, and Ben could always find a way to make his little son laugh. As he stretched out a foot to touch Melissa's ankle, Ben also realized that spending time with his family had inspired new love and respect for his wife in her role as nurturing mother. Their shared experience had brought them closer, despite the difficult times when all they wanted to do was sleep. *Jacob's a lucky kid*, he told himself. *Two parents who are so different but who love their son, each in their own way.* And when Ben rolled over and saw his smiling, healthy baby in his wife's arms, he knew he was as lucky as his son.

CHAPTER 12

Weaning Your Baby

*"At nineteen months, my daughter is down to nursing only once
or twice per day. Soon she'll have weaned herself completely,
and I'll miss that part of our relationship when it's gone. I
am happy, however, that I chose to breastfeed my daughter, and
I can tell in her smile and her demeanor that she is, too!"*

—Erika, 27, mother of Charlotte

"Mommy, look!" Michelle, age two, called to her mother from
the top of the toddler slide on the neighborhood playground.
Gwen, her mother, waved from where she sat on a nearby bench,
chatting with her best friend, Susan. As the two women watched,
Michelle slid to the ground, shrieking with delight, and landed
with a plop at the bottom. Unfortunately, she bumped the back
of her head on the edge of the slide and ran to her mother, crying.

"Oh, Michie, that hurt, huh?" Gwen said, hurrying over to
pick up her crying toddler. "Poor Michelle. But it wasn't too bad,
was it? Want to come sit with Mama for a bit?" Gwen rejoined her
friend on the bench, cuddling Michelle on her lap and preparing
her for a comforting nursing session. But Michelle had already
wiped her tears from her eyes and wanted to get down. "Slide!"
she said, jumping off her mother's lap. A moment later she was
happily climbing the ladder again.

Gwen sighed. "Well, there she goes," she said to her friend.
"She hardly ever seems to want to nurse anymore, even when
she's upset."

"That's funny," Susan said, glancing over at the sandbox,

where her own two-year-old was playing. "Tina's barely slowed down at all. Fred and I decided when I was pregnant that I'd breastfeed until her second birthday if that's what Tina wanted, but that was three months ago and she still wants to nurse."

IS THIS GOOD-BYE?

The decision to stop breastfeeding is a personal choice, and many mothers are surprised that their own goals and desires in this area differ markedly from those of other mothers and even from those of their children. You may so enjoy the closeness that comes with breastfeeding that you want to continue nursing through toddlerhood. Your child may want to continue nursing long past his first year, particularly before bedtime and when he's in need of comfort. On the other hand, you may feel the need to move on to new activities, or your child's active temperament may cause him to be too impatient to continue to nurse. Whenever and for whatever reason you and your child decide that the time has come (or, as is sometimes the case, suddenly realize that feedings have tapered off almost of their own accord), look at this change as another positive step in your life together and a window into the fascinating new ways your child is growing.

IS THIS THE RIGHT TIME? WHEN TO WEAN

Planning ahead when to stop breastfeeding—or trying to decide what the best age for weaning might be—can be a particularly difficult exercise for parents in this country. Few, if any, cultural conventions tell us precisely when it's time to completely wean from the breast, yet concerned relatives and friends often seem to have strong opinions about what's best for the child and mother. The American Academy of Pediatrics recommends continued breastfeeding beyond the first birthday as long as mutually desired by mother and child. However, mothers in the United

An Experience of a Lifetime

COMMON FEELINGS ABOUT WEANING

Breastfeeding mothers' feelings about ending this period of their lives are as varied and intense as any other basic parenting experience. You may be surprised at how powerful and even turbulent your emotional response is to the idea of weaning your baby—whether you can hardly imagine no longer nursing or long for greater freedom. Some mothers may feel sad about giving up the closeness that comes from breastfeeding. Others may feel ambivalence between desire for greater independence from their babies and a longing for continued closeness.

Whatever your feelings about this major transition (and you may well experience all of them at one time or another), understand that such emotional responses are quite common and natural. By cuddling and interacting with your baby even more during the weaning process, you will start to stabilize your own emotions and adjust to this new stage in your life as a mother. Talk with friends who have experienced weaning with their own children or write down your own experiences to share with your child when she's grown. Finally, remember that weaning is a natural step in helping your child grow up. You will both make it through this transition and thrive as you find new ways to remain close.

States have tended to wean much earlier over the past century than in most other countries, paralleling the more widespread use of infant formula. Today, though, later weaning is steadily gaining wider acceptance in the general population. In addition, weaning is more often initiated by the mother in this country, whereas in most other cultures children begin the process when they feel ready. Worldwide, the average age for weaning is between two and four, and in some societies breastfeeding continues up to age six or seven.

Scientific research on the benefits of long-term breastfeeding for the health and well-being of child and mother is growing. Researchers have found that the composition of the mother's breastmilk continues to change during her baby's second year of life, and it continues to provide important nutritional benefits and to bolster the toddler's immune system. Studies have also demonstrated evidence of a "dose effect" for breastfeeding—meaning that the longer breastfeeding continues and the more breastmilk a child consumes, the better the health for child and mother. Further research has shown that the longer children are breastfed in their first year of life, the better they perform in tests of cognitive skills and academic achievement. This especially holds true for children who are breastfed for more than eight months. For these and many other reasons, the World Health Organization recommends exclusive breastfeeding for six months and urges mothers to continue breastfeeding at least until age two.

The simplest, most "natural" time to wean is when your child initiates the process. Weaning begins naturally at six months, when iron-fortified solid foods are introduced. Some children begin to turn gradually away from breastfeeding and toward other forms of nutrition and comfort at around one year of age, when they have begun to enjoy a wide variety of solid foods and have learned to drink from a cup. Others wean themselves during the toddler years as they become more physically active and less willing to sit still to nurse. Gradually tapering off the number of nursing sessions at this time can proceed quite smoothly, as your child becomes so busy with new experiences that she "forgets" that it's time to nurse.

You may, however, decide to initiate weaning at an earlier time for reasons of your own. These may include the need to be away from home for longer periods, a new pregnancy, job constraints, or even an increasing lack of desire to breastfeed. (It is important to remember, though, that you *can* continue to breastfeed even if you have become pregnant or return to work, perhaps reducing the frequency of breastfeeding and incorporating some use of infant formula.) Starting the weaning process yourself will not be as easy as following your child's lead, but with care and sensitivity it can certainly be accomplished. Meanwhile,

Weaning begins naturally around six months of age, when iron-fortified solid foods are introduced.

it's important to focus on your child's needs and your own—to tune out the inevitable advice and judgment of others outside the mother–child relationship, resist comparing your situation to

To Wean or Not to Wean

WHEN PARENTS DISAGREE

Many mothers—particularly those breastfeeding their first babies—are surprised at how much family tradition, cultural background, and the opinions of others come into play as they

consider the optimal time for weaning. As fathers in this
country become more involved in the parenting process in
general, they are also likely to have opinions—sometimes
quite strong ones—about when breastfeeding is appropriate
and at what age it is not. If your child's father comes from a
family whose traditions favor breastfeeding into toddlerhood,
he may disapprove of your desire to stop breastfeeding at,
say, your child's first birthday. If his own mother did not
breastfeed or clearly disapproves of your continuing to nurse,
he may pressure you to wean sooner than you or your baby
would like.

When facing such a situation, it is necessary to recognize
the father's desire to "do the right thing" for you and your
child and to appreciate the powerful forces that affect his
opinion. If you feel that his decisions on the matter spring
more from the sense that "that's the way it has always been
done" rather than from conclusions based on scientific evidence and expert advice, suggest that he read this book and
ask your pediatrician or La Leche League volunteer (see
Chapter 3) to refer you to a parenting group or fathers' club
that addresses this issue in the context of general child development. Finally, listen carefully to the reasons he gives for his
opinions. The final decision of when to wean should remain
with you and your child, but by focusing on Dad's issues and
finding other ways to satisfy his goals (allowing for more
time for him and his baby between nursing sessions, for in-
stance), you can turn this conflict into an opportunity for
growth and greater understanding for the entire family. If
conflict persists, consult your pediatrician or family physician
for additional help.

that of any other family, and maybe even rethink any advance deadlines you set for yourself when you were pregnant or your child was a newborn. Keep in mind that you have provided the best start for your baby by breastfeeding, no matter how early or late you decide to stop. Some breastfeeding is better than none. No one but you and your child can decide what is best for the two of you.

A GRADUAL PARTING: HOW TO WEAN

As indicated previously, weaning is a natural process, and it's best for you and your child if it happens in a natural way. The key word in this context is *gradual*—a gradual move toward other forms of nutrition and closeness, with the number and length of breastfeeding sessions tapering off over weeks or even months. In this way, you and your child will have time to find other ways to maintain closeness, express and accept tenderness or comfort, and ensure proper nutritional intake before you completely stop nursing. You will also avoid the conflicts and resistance that tend to spring from more abrupt weaning and even minimize your own physical difficulties such as breast engorgement.

Exposing a child to new foods during a regular breastfeeding time may help him wean.

One of the most effective ways to begin a gradual weaning process with a child age one or older is simply not to offer a feeding and wait to see if he requests it. The easiest first session to skip in this way is usually the midday breastfeeding, when your child may already have had access to a lunch of solid food and such liquids as cow's milk or fruit juice. Your child may well become so interested in another activity after lunch that he forgets about nursing and never requests a midday feeding again. If your child does signal a desire to nurse, however, be sure to satisfy his desire. In weaning, as in all developmental processes, it's best to follow your child's lead. In any case, refusing to breastfeed will only increase his desire and focus his attention on the activity. Distracting him with new foods or different kinds of interaction during his usual breastfeeding time is a more positive and effective way to help him wean.

Once your child has grown accustomed to missing the midday nursing session, take a look at skipping a second feeding in the same understated manner. Again, redirecting his attention to new activities, food options, and sources of emotional reassurance (such as a favorite blanket or stuffed animal) will help him make the transition more easily. If he decides that he wants to

A Healthy Substitute

INSTEAD OF BREASTMILK . . .

Your child's age is important in determining what kinds of nourishment to offer in place of breastmilk during the weaning process. Babies under age one should receive iron-fortified formula, not whole cow's milk. Children aged one to two can have whole milk. Reduced-fat milk, either low fat or skim, is appropriate for children aged two and older who are drinking cow's milk.

Not Quite Yet . . .

WHEN NOT TO WEAN

In most cases, the decision to wean can be based on a mother's and child's inner needs and practical considerations relating to the family. However, it's best to put off weaning in some situations until a time when conditions are better. Such situations include:

Food allergies. If you or your child's father have experienced food allergies, talk with your child's pediatrician or other health professional about the benefits of delaying weaning until at least after your child's first birthday. As pointed out in Chapter 7, avoiding cow's milk or cow's milk–based products may be helpful.

Illness. If your child has a cold, is teething, has recently been hospitalized, or is otherwise not in tip-top shape, put off initiating the weaning process until he feels better. You might also want to delay your first attempts if you feel under the weather. It's always best to meet any transition period when you and your child are at your physical and emotional best.

Changes at home. If you are pregnant or have recently had a new baby, this may not be the best time to wean, unless led by your child. On the other hand, your needs and the needs of a newborn may take priority. Always breastfeed the newborn first, but try to be sensitive to the needs of everyone involved. Likewise, a move to a new home, a marital disruption, a new child-care situation, your return to work, and other potentially stressful situations are not the best times to initiate another major change. Ideally, you will begin weaning when it's not overly stressful for you or your child.

nurse, offer the breast—thus reassuring him that you are still there for him as he continues to explore his surroundings. If he clings to one or two favorite feeding times—usually the last one before bedtime and the first one in the morning—consider continuing these sessions for as long as he wants to nurse. Such quiet times rarely interfere with even the busiest family's schedule and are a wonderful way to maintain that special closeness with your child.

Some mothers find that it is not so much the transition to other activities that challenges young children in the midst of the weaning process but the difficulty of adapting to new feeding methods such as a bottle or a cup. This is particularly true of infants and younger toddlers. In Chapter 9, methods to help your baby make the transition from breastfeeding to drinking expressed breastmilk from a cup or bottle were presented. The same methods can be used to move your child toward formula (if he is less than one year old) or milk (age one and older) during weaning. Keep in mind, though, that if you choose to wean your child to a bottle, you will have to wean to a cup later on. For best dental hygiene and to prevent tooth decay, babies older than one year of age should drink from a cup instead of a bottle.

You can use the same gradual method of substitution when introducing a younger baby to a bottle or cup as you would with an older child. If you decide to use a bottle, introduce it gradually over several days. Use it with one feeding—probably the midday session—and work your way up to more. It helps if your baby is not extremely hungry, because then he may be more patient when trying out the bottle. Pay attention to your baby's responses. Some breastfed babies accept a bottle more easily if someone other than the mother offers it. (But some prefer taking a bottle while in their mother's arms.) If you or another adult have tried for several days to get your baby to accept a bottle and he has continued to refuse, try changing to a different kind of nipple for a few days or switch to a cup. If your baby uses a pacifier, he may prefer a similar nipple for feedings. Babies can be particular about the type of nipple they use, but once they are introduced to one they like they may adjust easily. Meanwhile, during this learning process, don't force your baby to take a bottle. The process of bottle-feeding is quite different from breast-feeding, and his adjustment may well take time. Excess pressure to take a bottle may cause him to refuse the bottle (see Chapter 9).

After bottle-feedings have started, some babies get frustrated when nursing, because the milk doesn't flow as fast from the breast as from the bottle. If this is the case with your child, try offering him the breast before he gets too hungry and is too impatient to adapt to its naturally slower flow. Help your milk flow faster by massaging the breast as you nurse. (Pumping for one or two minutes before starting to breastfeed can start your milk flowing faster too.) A bottle with a slow-flowing nipple may also help diminish the difference between the bottle-feeding and breastfeeding experience.

Many mothers, particularly those whose babies are older, prefer to wean directly to a cup—thus eliminating the need to wean their child from the bottle later on. (A bottle can become a beloved security object for a child aged one or older, and persuading him to give it up can turn into quite a challenge.) To introduce your baby to a cup, start with a small plastic one or, even better, a trainer cup with a snap-on lid to prevent spills and two handles for your baby to grasp. Don't be surprised if he treats the cup as a toy at first. He will probably throw it nearly as

A trainer cup with a snap-on lid prevents spills if you choose to wean your child directly to a cup.

often as he drinks from it. This is perfectly normal baby or toddler behavior and part of the process of familiarizing himself with this new tool.

It is often the case when raising children that our best-laid parenting plans are disrupted by the realities of our particular children's personalities, needs, and situations. Even when you have made the time and taken care to proceed with weaning in a leisurely manner, your child may elect to cut down nursing quite abruptly or stop breastfeeding altogether. His desire to make this transition today instead of tomorrow is in no way a rejection of you but a sign of his independence. Likewise, if your child continues to need to nurse for longer than you had planned, do not interpret this as a sign that he is immature, lacks self-confidence,

● ✛ ◆ ✛ ● ✛ ◆ ✛ ● ✛ ◆ ✛ ● ✛

Slow Down!

PHYSICAL CHANGES DURING WEANING

When weaning is accomplished gradually, mothers of older babies and toddlers sometimes hardly notice at first that their milk has diminished and that other changes are taking place. One of the most important physical changes to note as your child moves from exclusive breastfeeding toward partial breastfeeding with the addition of formula, cow's milk, or solids is the gradual return of your hormones to their pre-pregnancy state. This is associated with normal cycling of your estrogen and progesterone levels, with release of eggs and the possibility of becoming pregnant. This possibility increases naturally after the baby reaches six months. Should you not want to become pregnant again right away, discuss alternate methods of birth control with your gynecologist and your partner (refer to Chapter 6 for a discussion of these methods), and be sure to begin using some type of birth control immediately.

Changes in your breasts will take place more gradually, even in cases when the weaning process itself moves at a brisk pace. You may continue to produce some milk for months—or even years—after your child has stopped nursing, particularly if your nipples continue to be stimulated or you otherwise check to see whether milk is still present. It will also probably take several months for your breasts to return to their pre-pregnancy size. After weaning, some women find that their breasts are slightly different in size or firmness than before their pregnancy. You should continue to perform monthly breast self-examinations throughout breastfeeding, including the weaning period, and bring any concerns about lumps or firmness to your doctor's attention.

Breast pain caused by engorgement should not be a problem if you are proceeding with weaning gradually. Your breasts will simply slow down milk production as demand decreases until little is produced and finally none. If your child has elected to stop nursing more abruptly, however, you may experience some discomfort. If this is the case, express just enough milk to keep your breasts from feeling so full—but keep in mind that expressing more than a small amount of breastmilk will spur greater milk production and increase discomfort even more. (Persistent, unrelieved engorgement may increase your risk of developing mastitis, an infection and/or inflammation of the breast.) Meanwhile, try to encourage your child to wean more gradually, if possible. You don't want to force him to breastfeed if he's not interested, of course, but slowing down the weaning pace a bit could make the process more comfortable for you. This process may also signal that your little one is ready to move on to a new stage in your relationship.

or is overly dependent on you. Instead, you can be reassured that your child still values breastfeeding sessions and receives security and comfort from cuddling during nursing.

IF YOUR CHILD RESISTS

Some children strongly object to their mother's efforts to move from breast- to bottle- or cup-feeding, no matter how sensitively and gradually the process is approached. This resistance can become frustrating if you want or need to wean by a specific time (for example, if you need to start back to work or school and have decided not to express your breastmilk during your separation). Unfortunately, the more anxious you become about completing the weaning process, the more difficult it may become as

Your toddler may turn to nursing for comfort and reassurance but will still receive nutritional and immunologic benefits.

your baby picks up on your feelings of impatience. The best approach is to take a deep breath, remember that "this too shall pass," and review the previous section for additional advice. Consider shortening your nursing sessions as a prelude to dropping them altogether. At the times of day when your child is used to nursing, stay away from your usual nursing locations, involve her in an interesting activity, and avoid such strong nursing cues as pulling her onto your lap, uncovering your breasts in front of her, or even sitting down. Don't forget to offer her even more than the usual amount of affection, hugs, and kisses, though. The emotional component of breastfeeding is powerful for the older baby and toddler and is best replaced with other forms of physical contact and expressions of your love.

If your baby still resists, consider whether you might continue breastfeeding—just less often—while offering a cup, bottle, or other foods at other times. By partially weaning (for example, initially keeping the early-morning and before-bed feedings, and then gradually dropping the early-morning session), you eliminate a source of conflict between your child and yourself that may turn out to be unnecessary. You also send your child the message that you are paying attention to her feelings and responding to them. Eventually, you can agree with your older child on an endpoint for nursing. In the meantime, your willingness to recognize her needs and provide for them sets an excellent pattern in your relationship for the years to come.

PLAY WITH ME! A NEW RELATIONSHIP WITH YOUR CHILD

Michelle was now nearly three, still active, and fully weaned. Her mother, Gwen, smiled with pride as she watched her race a little boy across the playground. Over the past six months, Gwen had recognized the fact that her naturally adventurous daughter now preferred playing to nursing. (In fact, she felt that breastfeeding had contributed to Michelle's exuberance, self-confidence, and

Q & A
Does She Still Need Me?

Q: *I have just learned that I must have surgery a week from now. I'm afraid that breastfeeding will be too difficult during my recovery, and I'm thinking about weaning over the next seven days. Can I wean my baby in such a short time?*

A: As noted in Chapter 5, few types of surgery require a woman to stop breastfeeding entirely. In cases that require a temporary interruption in breastfeeding, consider expressing breastmilk before the surgery and freezing it for your baby's use until you can resume nursing. Abrupt weaning should be attempted only when no alternative presents itself. If you must end breastfeeding in a brief time, try following the steps laid out in the previous sections of this chapter, but speed them up somewhat. Apply cabbage leaves to your breasts to ease your discomfort (see page 149). Your child may resist the accelerated pace, but you will at least have introduced her to alternative feeding possibilities before you wean completely. Be sure to make time for a great deal of cuddling, playing, and other non-nursing-related contact to cushion any feelings of confusion your child may experience. Meanwhile, keep in mind your own need to adjust to this sudden change by easing breast engorgement (see above) and making allowances for hormonal and emotional fluctuations.

Q: *My toddler seems to get most of his calories from solid foods and cow's milk and wants to breastfeed only when he's upset or tired. Is it healthy to continue breastfeeding if nursing has turned into a comfort ritual more than anything else?*

A: Your toddler may turn to nursing for comfort and reassurance, but he is certainly still benefiting from the nutritional and immunologic benefits. In any case, emotional support is a perfectly legitimate aspect of breastfeeding. Seeking out a reassuring nursing session when he's upset and bouncing back as soon as he finishes builds your child's confidence and feelings of security and well-being. Certainly there is no evidence that extended breastfeeding makes a child more dependent or harms him in any way. On the contrary, many parents proudly tell how independent, healthy, and exceptionally bright their long-term breastfed children become. As long as you are comfortable breastfeeding your toddler, there is no reason to stop.

Q: *My three-year-old is nearly weaned but still has a hard time falling asleep without nursing. Is it okay to nurse her to sleep, or should I insist that she learn to fall asleep on her own?*

A: Falling asleep at the breast is a profoundly satisfying experience for a young child—one she has probably enjoyed from her earliest days. While it is true that children need to explore different ways to let go of wakefulness at the end of the day, a nursing session just before bedtime can help your daughter relax enough to focus on this skill and succeed at it. Since any kind of milk or juice can promote tooth decay when in contact with your baby's teeth for long periods, try offering your child the breast just before brushing her teeth and then ease her toward sleep with a bedtime story and a kiss good-night.

independence.) Of course, Gwen loved the closeness that feeding had provided. She even felt an occasional pang of envy when she saw her friend, Susan, settle down for one of the two or three daily nursing sessions that her daughter still enjoyed. Still, as Michelle made one of her routine detours toward her mother for a quick word of praise and a hug, Gwen noted that she and her daughter had found new ways to relate that reflected their expanding understanding of each other's needs and desires. Breastfeeding was one of the most meaningful times of Gwen's life, and she looked forward to having the same relationship with all her future children. But she also knew that she and her daughter had a world of experiences ahead of them. She had no doubt that Michelle would enjoy them all to the fullest, since she'd had such an excellent start.

You, too, can congratulate yourself on a job well done as you complete this stage of your breastfeeding relationship with your child. Being a nursing mother takes a tremendous amount of knowledge, effort, and time, but it is also one of the most rewarding experiences a mother can have. As you watch your baby grow into a healthy, confident, secure child, you will see those first lessons in love and commitment take root and enhance his ability to make friends and communicate with others. Someday, when he is a parent with his own newborn to care for, you will be able to remind him how his life started and second his conviction that nature's gift for babies is the best gift of all.

APPENDIX I

BREASTFEEDING RESOURCES

Academy of Breastfeeding Medicine
191 Clarksville Road
Princeton Junction, NJ 08550
(877) 836-9947
http://www.bfmed.org
The Academy of Breastfeeding Medicine is an international organization of physicians with expertise or interest in breastfeeding research, education, and support.

Baby Friendly, USA
8 Jan Sebastian Way # 22
Sandwich, MA 02563
(508) 888-8092
http://www.babyfriendlyusa.org
The Baby Friendly Hospital Initiative is an international program of the World Health Organization (WHO) and the United Nations Children's Fund (UNICEF). Based on the WHO/ UNICEF *Ten Steps to Successful Breastfeeding,* the Initiative recognizes hospitals and birth centers that have taken steps to provide an optimal environment for the promotion, protection, and support of breastfeeding. Baby Friendly, USA, is the organization that oversees implementation of the Baby Friendly Hospital Initiative in the United States.

*Please note: Website information, addresses, and phone numbers are subject to change.

Centers for Disease Control and Prevention
1600 Clifton Rd.
Atlanta, GA 30333
Public Inquiries
(404) 639-3311
(800) 311-3435
http://www.cdc.gov/
The Centers for Disease Control and Prevention (CDC) provides
resources and education in the area of illness, infectious diseases,
and health promotion.

Cleft Line
104 South Estes Dr., Suite 204
Chapel Hill, NC 27514
(800) 242-5338
The Cleft Line provides referral to a local support group for
parents of babies with facial birth defects.

Doulas of North America (DONA)
P.O. Box 626
Jasper, IN 47547
(888) 788-DONA
http://www.dona.org/
DONA can help you locate a doula in your area.

Human Milk Banking Assn. of North America
c/o Mothers' Milk Bank
WakeMed
3000 New Bern Ave.
Raleigh, NC 27610
(919) 350-8599
This organization provides guidance and policies regarding the
collection, storage, processing, and use of human milk.

International Board of Lactation Consultant Examiners (IBLCE)
7309 Arlington Blvd., Suite 300
Falls Church, VA 22042-3215
(703) 560-7330
http://www.iblce.org/
IBLCE oversees the process of examination and certification of
lactation consultants.

International Lactation Consultant Assn. (ILCA)
1500 Sunday Dr., Suite 102
Raleigh, NC 27607
(919) 787-5181
http://www.ilca.org/
ILCA is the professional organization of lactation consultants and
may be able to provide assistance with locating a lactation
consultant in your area.

La Leche League International, Inc.
1400 North Meacham Rd.
Schaumburg, IL 60173-4048
(847) 519-7730
(800) LaLeche
http://www.lalecheleague.org/
La Leche League International provides a directory of volunteer
personnel who coordinate the activities of local groups, as well
as a comprehensive Website with current information about
breastfeeding, a catalog of publications and additional breastfeeding resources, and guides to international meetings and
breastfeeding seminars for health-care professionals. See local
phone listings to locate meetings in your area.

National Organization of Mothers of Twins Club
Executive Office
P. O. Box 438
Thompson Station, TN 37179-0438
(615) 595-0936 or (877) 540-2200
http://www.nomotc.org/
This organization is a network of nearly 500 clubs representing
parents of twins, triplets, and quadruplets. It fosters development
of local support groups, participates in research projects, and will
put you in touch with local chapters.

Nursing Mothers Counsel, Inc.
P. O. Box 50063
Palo Alto, CA 94303
(408) 291-8008
http://www.nursingmothers.org
The Nursing Mothers Counsel provides information and
publications on breastfeeding for mothers and health-care
professionals.

Wellstart International
P.O. Box 80877
San Diego, CA 92138-0877
(619) 295-5192
http://www.wellstart.org
Wellstart International promotes breastfeeding on a local,
national, and international level by training and equipping
health-care professionals and developing breastfeeding
curriculum, materials, and policy.

WIC: Special Supplemental Nutrition Program for Women,
Infants, and Children
http://www.fns.usda.gov/wic/CONTENT/BF/brpromo.htm
The goals of the National Breastfeeding Promotion Campaign of
WIC are to encourage participants to begin and to continue
breastfeeding by increasing referrals to WIC for breastfeeding
support, increasing public acceptance and support of
breastfeeding, and providing support and technical assistance to
WIC state and local professionals in the promotion of
breastfeeding. Consult local phone listings for offices in your area
or call the local health department.

National WIC Association
2001 S St. NW, Suite 580
Washington, DC 20009
(202) 232-5492
http://www.wicdirectors.org

BOOKS TO SHARE WITH CHILDREN

I Eat at Mommy's, Anna E. Bradley-McBeth
Will There Be a Lap for Me?, Dorothy Corey
Maggie's Weaning, Mary Joan Deutschbein
About Twins, Shelly Rotner, Sheila M. Kelly
We Like to Nurse, Chia Martin
See How You Grow, Dr. Patricia Pearse
Michele, the Nursing Toddler, Jane M. Pinczuk
On Mother's Lap, Ann Herbert Scott
The Best Gifts, Marsha Forchuk Skrypuch
The Cuddlers, Stacy Towle-Morgan
A Baby Just Like Me, Susan Winter

APPENDIX 2

RESOURCES FROM THE AMERICAN ACADEMY OF PEDIATRICS

The American Academy of Pediatrics (AAP) develops and produces a wide variety of public education materials that teach parents and children the importance of preventive and therapeutic medical care. Some examples of these materials include:

- Brochures and fact sheets on a myriad of health and parenting issues, including allergies, child care, divorce and single parenting, growth and development, injury prevention, immunizations, learning disabilities, breastfeeding, nutrition and fitness, sleep problems, substance abuse prevention, and the media's influence on young people.
- Videos on immunizations, newborn care, nutrition education, and asthma.
- Child-care books for children in various age groups, including the first year of life, birth to 5, 5 to 12, and 12 to 21, as well as topic-specific titles addressing common symptoms, nutrition, sleep, asthma and allergies, and breastfeeding.
- First aid/choking and CPR chart.
- Informative Websites. The Academy's Website, at *www.aap.org*, answers questions about child health and also features information on all aspects of child rearing—from injury prevention to teen dating, fears and phobias to car-seat usage. All the information on this site has been reviewed and approved by the American Academy of Pediatrics and represents the collective wisdom of more than 55,000 pediatricians. Parents can also access consumer health information from the AAP at *www.medem.com*, an e-health network created by the AAP and other leading medical societies.

To keep current on new AAP public education materials, please visit the Websites listed above.

APPENDIX 3

BREASTFEEDING RECORD

Use this record when you breastfeed and when your baby needs a diaper change during the first week. This will help you keep track of how well your baby is breastfeeding. Look at the sample.

1. Circle the hour closest to when your baby starts each breast-feeding.
2. Circle the **W** when the baby has a wet diaper.
3. Circle the **BM** when the baby has a bowel movement.

It is okay for your baby to have more wet diapers or bowel movements than the goal. If your baby has less than the goal, call your pediatrician or lactation specialist.

● ✛ SAMPLE ✛ ◆	GOAL
①2③4 5⑥7 8⑨10⑪ noon 1②3④5 6⑦8 9⑩11 12	at least 8-12
Wet diapers Ⓦ	1
Bowel movements—black ⒷⓂ ⒷⓂ	1

On the first day the baby fed 9 times, wet 1 diaper and had 2 dirty diapers.

✦ ◆ BIRTHDAY ● ✦	GOAL
1 2 3 4 5 6 7 8 9 10 11 noon 1 2 3 4 5 6 7 8 9 10 11 12	at least 8-12
Wet diapers W	1
Bowel movements—black BM	1

● ✦ ONE DAY OLD ✦ ◆	GOAL
1 2 3 4 5 6 7 8 9 10 11 noon 1 2 3 4 5 6 7 8 9 10 11 12	at least 8-12
Wet diapers W W	2
Bowel movements—black BM BM	2

✦ ◆ TWO DAYS OLD ● ✦	GOAL
1 2 3 4 5 6 7 8 9 10 11 noon 1 2 3 4 5 6 7 8 9 10 11 12	at least 8-12
Wet diapers W W W	3
Bowel movements—green BM BM	2

● ✦ THREE DAYS OLD ✦ ◆	GOAL
	at least 8-12
1 2 3 4 5 6 7 8 9 10 11 noon 1 2 3 4 5 6 7 8 9 10 11 12	
Wet diapers W W W W	4
Bowel movements—yellow green	
BM BM BM	3

✦ ◆ FOUR DAYS OLD ● ✦	GOAL
	at least 8-12
1 2 3 4 5 6 7 8 9 10 11 noon 1 2 3 4 5 6 7 8 9 10 11 12	
Wet diapers W W W W W	5
Bowel movements—yellow BM BM BM	3

● ✦ FIVE DAYS OLD ✦ ◆	GOAL
	at least 8-12
1 2 3 4 5 6 7 8 9 10 11 noon 1 2 3 4 5 6 7 8 9 10 11 12	
Wet diapers W W W W W W	6
Bowel movements—yellow	
BM BM BM BM	4

SIX DAYS OLD	GOAL
1 2 3 4 5 6 7 8 9 10 11 noon 1 2 3 4 5 6 7 8 9 10 11 12	at least 8-12
Wet diapers W W W W W W	6-8
Bowel movements—yellow	
BM BM BM BM	4-12

DATE:	GOAL
1 2 3 4 5 6 7 8 9 10 11 noon 1 2 3 4 5 6 7 8 9 10 11 12	at least 8-12
Wet diapers W W W W W W	6-8
Bowel movements—yellow	
BM BM BM BM	4-12

DATE:	GOAL
1 2 3 4 5 6 7 8 9 10 11 noon 1 2 3 4 5 6 7 8 9 10 11 12	at least 8-12
Wet diapers W W W W W W	6-8
Bowel movements—yellow	
BM BM BM BM	4-12

DATE: ● ✛ ◆ ✛	GOAL
	at least
1 2 3 4 5 6 7 8 9 10 11 noon 1 2 3 4 5 6 7 8 9 10 11 12	8-12
Wet diapers W W W W W W	6-8
Bowel movements—yellow	
BM BM BM BM	4-12

DATE: ● ✛ ◆ ✛	GOAL
	at least
1 2 3 4 5 6 7 8 9 10 11 noon 1 2 3 4 5 6 7 8 9 10 11 12	8-12
Wet diapers W W W W W W	6-8
Bowel movements—yellow	
BM BM BM BM	4-12

DATE: ● ✛ ◆ ✛	GOAL
	at least
1 2 3 4 5 6 7 8 9 10 11 noon 1 2 3 4 5 6 7 8 9 10 11 12	8-12
Wet diapers W W W W W W	6-8
Bowel movements—yellow	
BM BM BM BM	4-12

APPENDIX 4
DIETARY GUIDELINES

What Counts as a Serving?	How many servings do you need each day?		
	1600 calories[*]	2200 calories[*]	2800 calories[*]
Bread, Cereal, Rice, and Pasta Group • 1 slice of bread • About 1 cup ready-to-eat cereal • ½ cup cooked cereal, rice, or pasta	6	9	11
Vegetable Group • 1 cup raw leafy vegetables • ½ cup other vegetables—cooked or raw • ¾ cup vegetable juice	3	4	5
Fruit Group • 1 medium apple, banana, orange, pear • ½ cup chopped, cooked, or canned fruit • ¾ cup fruit juice	2	3	4

Milk, Yogurt, and Cheese Group—
Preferably fat free or low fat
• 1 cup milk[***] or yogurt
• 1½ ounces natural cheese
  (such as cheddar)
• 2 ounces processed cheese
  (such as American)
	2 or 3[**]	2 or 3[**]	2 or 3[*]

Meat, Poultry, Fish, Dry Beans, Eggs,
and Nuts Group—preferably lean or low fat
• 2–3 ounces cooked lean meat,
    poultry, or fish
  These count as 1 ounce of meat:
• ½ cup cooked dry beans or tofu
• 2½ ounces soyburger
• 1 egg
• 2 tablespoons peanut butter
• ⅓ cup nuts
	2, for a total of
	5 ounces
		2, for a total of
		6 ounces
			3, for a total of
			7 ounces

[*] Recommended number of servings depends on your caloric needs:
- 1600 calories is about right for children ages 2 to 6 years, many sedentary women, and some older adults.
- 2200 calories is about right for most children over 6, teen girls, active women, and many sedentary men.
- 2800 calories is about right for teen boys and active men.

[**] Children and teens, ages 9 to 18 years, and adults over age 50 need 3 servings daily; others need 2 servings daily.

[***] This includes lactose-free and lactose-reduced milk products. Soy-based beverages with added calcium are an option for those who prefer a nondairy source of calcium.

NOTE: Many of the serving sizes given above are smaller than those on the Nutrition Facts Label. For example, 1 serving of cooked cereal, rice, or pasta is 1 cup on the label, but only ½ cup on the Pyramid.

Source, Using the Dietary Guidelines for Americans (consumer pamphlet), Dietary Guidelines for Americans, 2000, 5th edition, United States Department of Agriculture, Center for Nutrition Policy and Promotion.

INDEX

Boldfaced numbers indicate illustration.